The Healing of My Thirty-Six Years of Migraines for The Quality of Life!

DR JACK TAN

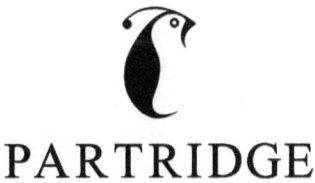

PARTRIDGE

ISBN: Hardcover   978-1-5437-6818-3
             Softcover   978-1-5437-6812-1
             eBook   978-1-5437-6817-6

To order additional copies of this book, contact
Toll Free +65 3165 7531 (Singapore)
Toll Free +60 3 3099 4412 (Malaysia)
orders.singapore@partridgepublishing.com

www.partridgepublishing.com/singapore

Contents

Preface

This book shares the treatments, healing processes, and recover journeys amidst difficulties of the author's migraine.

The author looked forward to conquer his severe migraine and to contribute to Singapore in asset management, banking and finance knowledge transfer through training programs and banking books with case studies illustrated by his experiences.

After 36 years, I, the author, have recovered from severe migraine. Since 1 February 1978, I had been in pain management and treatments of migraine attacks that occurred daily. fears from 1980. The banks' panel of doctors were not neurologists, but family doctors per se. After I resigned from the bank employed me because the migraine affected my right hand badly in which I could not type for five minutes, and the painful level was at level 10. I, the author, realised that I need to find a neurologist with specialist knowledge to healing of my migraine, commented by a friend to whom I knows.

My readers, you should never give up on seeking neurological treatments. You must trace the reasons of your case that suggested patients must know the internal and external factors. Aim to recover, no matter how tough it is! That should be your commitment to yourself and your family!

Suppose you suffer from migraine and want to find a solution to heal your headaches. You must know yourselves and seek a neurologist for treatments.

You have to manage your medical cost, career, and family towards treatments.

As a matter of protection and principle, never overdose, my dear readers.

You must know the risk factors while managing the fear factors psychologically if you have known them.

They are interrelated.

I was a fighter of migraine headaches for my benefit and family's protection with my loved career or business in which I recorded in my diaries to know migraine. Better.

Research shows that in the United States, about 85% of women, about twenty-three million of them, suffer from migraine. Study showed about one billion people world-wide suffer from migraines.

I regained the freedom of life from migraines and for the quality of life on 1 March 2014, healing me 8 years ago by Dr K Tan.

No more pain and insufferable migraine attacks since then! I am confident with my health until today! The agonising migraine I suffered was beyond imagination!

Despite my love of banking and finance career and contributions as a qualified trainer requested by the Singapore Central Bank's (also known as the MAS) Institute of Banking and Finance (IBF) from 1988 until March 2002 under the new charter for IBF became effective.

I recorded my migraine attacks' conditions, treatments, and pain management in a diary.

Acknowledgements

I acknowledge Dr K Tan's caring heart and exceptional knowledge of migraine and its neurological treatments and pain management.

I acknowledge the Singapore Central Bank's Institute of Banking and Finance (IBF). As a qualified trainer, they requested me to be a part-time lecturer. The bank employed me with the approval of its top management to help the Singapore Central Bank. I imparted my banking knowledge and skills through training programmes. Before its new charter, under the IBF, the participants of my training programmes, from 1988 until March 2002, are division heads, SVPs, VPs, AVPs, managers, and specialists. The mission was possible, and Singapore made it to the third or fourth spot as a global financial center.

I acknowledge those banks' doctors for treating my migraine, in one way or another, since 1978.

I thank Dr K Tan who listened intently and treated my migraine with patience and care for about 12 years. Dr K Tan healed my migraine entirely on 1 March 2014, and I stopped taking expensive migraine medicine – RELPAX (film-coated tablets, 40mg).

To allow me to have an entire understanding of migraine and its pain management, I read loads of books on fruits and vegetables that are not only rich in vitamin C but also antioxidants, which could help reduce the frequency of migraine occurrence for at least 36 years!

Friends and former colleagues who knew I was healed from migraine congratulated me and were so happy for me.

I gained quality of life, and free from migraines was my goal, on 1 March 2014 from 1 February 1978.

I completed and submitted my doctoral thesis on 9 August 2017 to the University of Western Australia with a doctorate degree in business administration (Tan, 2019).

Chapter 1

Introduction

What can you do to help manage your migraine?

A migraine is a severe pounding headache, and it can last for hours, if not days.

I do not have these situations from 1 February 1978 to 1 March 2014. The contributing factors should be unwelcoming stress although I loved my banking and finance career.

My migraine was without aura, but it was a daily event, and that was frightening because of fear factors developed psychologically.

There are several types of migraine (Karsan and Goadsby, 2018). I summaries them as follows:

Classic Migraine. It may be as complicated as migraines. The trigger point usually starts with a warning sign termed aura (Karsan and Goadsby, 2018). It is also referred as "migraine with aura."

Common Migraine (no aura). It may be called "migraine without aura." Common migraine can start slower than classic migraine. This migraine is without head pain and may be referred to as "silent migraine" (Karsan and Goadsby, 2018).

Hemiplegic Migraine. It's a symptom to cause one side of your body to become weak on either side (left or right) (Karsan and Goadsby, 2018). This is the type of migraine I had suffered for 36 years (from 1 February 1978 to 1 March 2014).

Retinal Migraine. They may also refer to ocular migraine and cause vision changes that are not aura vision changes (Karsan and Goadsby, 2018).

Ice-Pick Headaches. They are not migraine. They produce a stabbing pain around your eye and temples. It can be from either side, left or right, of the forehead. The author suffered from the right side of the body (Karsan and Goadsby, 2018).

Cluster Headaches. They are rare headaches. They occur in patterns, termed clusters (Karsan and Goadsby, 2018).

Cervicogenic Headaches. They are not migraine. They are headaches caused by another illness or physical condition; it could be a neck problem (Karsan and Goadsby, 2018).

Migraine is a neurological condition that can include a severe headache (Blau, J N; Dexter, S L; 1981) that may last for hours, sensitivity to light, aura, and vomiting. However, I did not have all these, except vomiting, twice over the 36 years (from 1 February 1978 to 1 March 2014). Dr K Tan healed my migraine.

I suffered a migraine attack on 1 February 1978, after joining my first loved career, banking, and finance on completing my National Service Obligations as a Commissioned Armed Forces Officer.

My migraine is with a stiffening right hand (Level 5 in Appendix 1); the symptoms are not kind to me. It constantly attacked my right side of the brain and eye, neck, and hand, turning into a stiff right hand at a pain level of 5 (Appendix 1).

I must quickly take migraine medicines to stop it and record them in my diaries. I had to face risk factors and fear factors, but I managed that so carefully!

The common symptoms of my migraine attacks are the following (Saper M D and Magee M D, 1981):

> Pain on the right side of the head
> Pain on the right eye
> Stiffness and aches on the right side of the neck
> Stiffness and aches on the right hand
> Vision difficulties
> Sensitivity to lights, sounds, and smells

I suffer the first four symptoms – stiff right hand, stiff and in pain right side of the neck, pain on the right eye, and pain on the right side of the head – if I do not take migraine medicines on time (Level 5 in Appendix 1) or quickly on its occurrence. I have a record in diaries of migraine attacks (the level of painfulness from level 1 to level 10). I measured level 5 symptoms. I must take medicines to stop migraine. My symptoms were recurring daily that created risk of overdosages (Appendix 1)., I was fearful and careful in consulting the bank's doctors from 1978 to 31 March 2002.

Record of the Level of Pain in Terms of Grade Representations in My Diary

I use the gradings to help me take medicines, Pons tan and Cafe got (Dr P Tang and various doctors from banks employed me, pain killers from 1978 to 2002). The neurological specialist doctor recommended that I must take ownership of finding the grading of pains coming to take RELPAX on time, not allowing the attack to manage it as protection. The doctor treated my migraine headaches from Dr K Tan in 2002 to 2022. I must discuss with Dr K. Tan that I want to keep my future appointment dates open because I am okay after my recovery on 1 March 2014.

1985 was an x-ray on my brain, but 1990 was an MRI on my brain at the government hospital. The results of the x-ray and MRI were showing my brain was fine and without evidence of any problems of tumours. The two technical analyses were all right that put me at ease and improved my confidence in healing my migraine attacks in 1985 and 1990 respectively, even though it was a daily occurrence. Those were costly even with the government's subsidies for pioneer patients like me, the first batch of National Service Male, contributed to r Singapore's defence.

Evidence

The cost for x-ray my brain in 1985 and the MRI in 1990 were necessary procedures because the doctors needed the evidence from technical analyses before otherwise (Note: explain here to you, Mr Emman, my editor.)

The second contribution was in the banking and finance sector despite my severe migraine illness (Dr K Tan's consultation, 2022).

The second contribution was in the banking and finance sector despite my severe migraine illness (Dr K Tan's consultation, 2022). It was Singapore Central Bank's decision for the ably experienced corporate banking senior to contribute the knowledge and skills.

Hence, Singapore Central Bank's (also known as the Monetary Authority of Singapore) Institute of Banking and

The Healing of My Thirty-Six Years of Migraines for The Quality of Life!

5

Finance requested me to contribute as a qualified trainer and part-time lecturer for imparting my knowledge, skills, and experience to banks' SVPs, VPs and AVPs, managers and specialists in structured trade finance and commodities financings and credit risk management through training programmes designed by me as a recognition.

The evidence refers to the strict requirements of getting Singapore as a global financial centre in the world, currently in a third or fourth position.

The syndications of loans involving aircraft financings and ship financings were under my care in the corporate banking division in the large Singapore bank before a foreign bank headhunted me to be head of corporate banking division doing syndications of loans on aircraft and aircraft engines financings and structured trade and commodities financings.

I started my banking and finance career on 1 February 1975 after being discharged from National Service obligations. My migraine was brought about by my job as head of import trade finance in the mid-size American bank after it completed the acquisition of a progressive bank in Hong Kong, which was short-handed, in 1978. Unfortunately, my migraine began to develop, and initially, the bank's doctor prescribed medicines like Aspirin and Panadol. In 1980, the frequency of migraine attacks did not decrease but increased.

By October 1980, a local bank invited me to join the bank's international division's import trade finance department. Even though my employment bank has medical benefits, I must visit the doctor for ordinary migraine. However, when I was referred for treatment to a neurologist in a private hospital, at Mt. Elizabeth Hospital's migraine clinic, I had to bear all costs myself. That cost was a bomb on my bills, adding stress in my financial position. Therefore, I saved about 20% from my income in addition to CPF contribution under the Singapore laws on CPF contributions.

Life and Healthcare

A person should live a healthy life so that the person can contribute to the country.

The author did not know if there was any correlation with his birth's diarrhoea illness. The author should thank his dear mum with respect. Without her care, the author might not have survived. There was a challenge growing up with the author and helping the author's father and mum in their spring sprouts business.

The author's father had high expectations from the author. The author's starting life was tough, but his endurance transformed him. He trained to be a tough person with a goal and two objectives (Dr Tan, 2021). Because of the dear mum and medical team's care, he survived under the extreme difficulty of growing up with diarrhoea at birth.

Life is the fact that the author must deal with.

Knowing the birth of diarrhoea illness may have relations to my migraine as a precaution. It was also evident that when my migraine attack was before I took the medicine, in those days were Pons tan and Cafe got. I would have to go toilet to pass motions and the migraine would subside within 20 minutes (1992 experiences recorded in my diaries.) That was from my personal experience. I could have the recollection that it happened three times over the 36 years of sufferings from my diaries.

I, the author, now keeps my life with a guided procedure and sufficient exercise to have a healthy body and reads daily.

Appendix 1

The pain level grading that helped me in pain management is as follows:

1   5   10

I was fearful that the migraine's vicious cycle was coming using the grading system to guide me in taking Pons tan and Cafe got medicines from 1980 until March 2002 under the strict disciple could not be ignored (Appendix 1).

Use a diary's calendar to record the migraine attack and the level of pains as a crystal sign and pain management

Month (for example - January 1978)

No	Su	Mo	Tu	We	Th	Fr	Sa
1	1 L-	2 L-5 (RN, 9:30am)	3 L-	4 L-	5 L-	6 L-	7 L-
2	8 L-	9 L-	10 L-	11 L-	12 L-	13 L-	14 L-
3	15 L-	16 L-	17 L-	18 L-	19 L-	20 L-	21 L-
4	22 L-	23 L-	24 L-	25 L-	26 L-	27 L-	28 L-
5	29 L-	30 L-	31 L-				

Note: L = Level of gradings (Self-invented to have control management)

For example, on 2 January 1978, Monday at 9:30am, my right neck became stiff, and the level was 5. That was before 1 February 1978. The progressive worsening of migraine is cumulated and a sign of getting negative results. The reader(s) should refer to the summary in my diary calendar. I managed the method for 36 years until Dr K Tan healed me in a government hospital recommended by my friend in April 2002 (Chapter 8). The daily episodes made me so fearful and record the event of attacks, but I fought on against the evil migraine.

What does a migraine attack mean to me?

Migraine is a symptomatically heterogeneous condition, and headache may be one manifestation (Karsan and Goadsby, 2018). No one can stand the pains from migraine headaches on the forehead, eye, hand, and neck on either side – right or left side of the body, including typing with a hand at the computer on my banking works, neck, eye, and brain (Karsan and Goadsby, 2018).

Back in my pre-university (now A levels) days in 1968, I recollected that each time I went to the cinema, I had a mild headache after the show. That was a crystal-clear sign that I could not go to crowded places and that I needed fresh air. Also, my weakest points were on the right side of my body – hand, neck, head, and eye. I followed a strict self-disciple to prevent getting migraine attacks under my preventive governance. That is for me, family, and health. Thus, exercising is my routine for management of my healthy body now. I jog about 5 KMs on each other days.

Headache is a prevalent symptom and may be collectively headache disorder (Ahmed, 2019; Karsan and Goadsby, 2018).

The stiffness and pains (forehead, eye, hand, and neck) mostly occurred on my right side, but some patients may feel it on the left side of the body.

My right hand is always stiff after typing credit proposals for long hours. My doctor suggested that I rest after sitting in front of the computer typing credit analyses or guiding relationship managers. To increase my productivity, doctors I consulted advised me to take a break every half an hour and not sit in front of the computer for more than one hour. Thus, I developed the discipline of time management.

When I sit in my office doing my corporate banking credit analyses and deals for a few hours, it may trigger stiffness on my right hand, a symptom signifying that the migraine attack is developing and coming. My doctor recommended that I set the grades from 1 to 10 (Appendix 1) as measurements and record in diaries. The supervision of all relationship managers needed skills and knowledge of corporate banking services and structuring of credit facilities for potential borrowers. Sharing knowledge is a vital part of relationship-building. It is crucial that the credit committee effortlessly understands the power of risk analysis and structure of credit facilities.

Duke-NUS Medical School and Novartis Singapore Pte Ltd released new findings from a study on 18 September 2019 (Ong et al., 2019). The research found that migraine places a substantial economic burden (S$1.04 billion in 2018) on Singapore (Ong et al., 2019) and the sufferers' quality of life and fears.

Hence, I was careful about a venue that must not be too crowded because I needed fresh air as the first line of defence to prevent the occurrence of migraine. Life went on, and looking back, when I was performing my National Service obligations in military field training, I was all right even though it was under the hot sun. It did not affect me because field training in the open space has a lot of fresh air. However, I was only worried about my parents' work in the spring sprouts business. Likewise, when I was in university, I worried about my parents' company in the spring sprouts business.

I know my reasons for having migraine. I was sensitive to crowded places that lacked fresh air.

Some of the trigger points of my migraine headaches in those days, apart from sitting posture in front of my computer typing credit proposal(s) for the secured deals or recommending that my relationship managers improve the credit proposal(s) for the Credit Committee meeting on Monday.

I restricted myself to half an hour typing at the computer for my work as suggested by my doctors. I took a five-minute walk that would not affect my productivity but instead would improve my blood circulation and prevent stiffness to the right side of my body – hand, neck, forehead, eye – because of long working hours.

Migraine and Foods and Fruits

I must avoid certain foods or fruits, including cheese and products with cheese elements, such as cheesecakes. So, I only loved foods or fruits that were suitable for me.

I must have enough rest and sound sleep after a day's work. I avoid red wine and alcohol. They were not for me. Hence, I had the strictest self-discipline and diets. I read loads of books, from banking and corporate finance books to storybooks to learn creative and pleasurable ways to relax my brain.

My migraine attacks started on 1 February 1978. We had heavy loads of bank work because we were short-handed. I suffered migraine for 36 years until I switched to a neurologist at a government hospital, Dr K Tan. He healed me on 1 March 2014, during my doctorate study and doctoral thesis writing at the University of Western Australia.

However, I loved my asset management investments company after banking and finance and training bank talents in the region, including Indonesian and Malaysian banks, People's Bank of China (Central Bank), and Taiwan's Central Bank's Research Academy and Banks in Hong Kong and Singapore at the Singapore government and the World Bank's requests.

My migraine headaches might have added a psychological fear on me while managing pains to reduce presenteeism (lower productivity) or avoid absenteeism (sick leave) always during the thirty-six years of migraine headache attacks. Thus, my good friend recommended me to a government hospital's neurologist. That was an appropriate decision, leading to my recovery of migraine on 1 March 2014.

People who suffer from migraine have worries and low quality of life. They are also under stress, in pain, and dependent on medicines. I suffered from migraine attacks until I was treated by Dr K Tan, a government hospital neurologist, and fully recovered. Thanks to Dr K Tan!

My goal was freedom of life transformation, giving me the quality of life and banking and finance and asset management investment career!

Dr K Tan freed me from migraine after treating me for about 12 years from about April 2002.

In summary, as a preventive action, I was careful about foods, liquids, biscuits, and fruits that I eat and/or must avoid. I read loads of books, in English and Chinese, on migraine. But

my discipline is that I must have enough rest after work. Every
night, when I returned from work, I had to spend time talking
to my dear mum as she was getting older. It was to ensure my
beloved mum was all right. Each year her friends were leaving
her, passing on.

In all, I have always kept a psychological balance for the
sake of avoiding migraine attacks. I recorded the occurrence of
migraine attacks in my diaries. How do I do it? I read the side
effects of RELPAX as opposed to the side effects of Pons tan
and Cafe got.

Going back to August 1992, I visited the bank that
employed me in corporate banking, doing structured financings
like syndications of loans on aircraft financing and other
structuring commodities financings. The doctor who treated
me was on annual leave. The relief doctor asked me to wait
until she finished reading my records. When she called me in,
she said, "You are still alive?"

"Of course," I said. "I do a lot of jogging, at least 6 km each
run, every other day."

That might have detoxifications in the process. Could it
be that detoxification helped me get rid of toxins, side effects?

She explained to me the side effects of Pons tan and Cafe
got. Of course, I was fearful of migraine medicines because of
the side effects.

The final one was only RELPAX after the private hospital's
pain management doctor suggested getting rid of Pons tan and
Cafe got. The doctor offered an expensive procedure, a few
thousand dollars for four days of hospital treatment, to stop my
dependency on Pons tan and Cafe got medicines.

But it was not successful. The pains management doctor
introduced me to RELPAX (expensive!) to get out of Pons tan
and Cafe got. I was semi-happy because no more Pons tan and

Cafe got, but I must now take RELPAX as a substitute. It was costly.

A friend recommended a neurologist in a government hospital to treat me. with a pioneer status get a subsidy.

Dr K Tan is soft-spoken, listened intently, and prescribed me with preventive medicines for migraine. I asked Dr K Tan to stop the preventive medication for migraine as they did not work on me. After the treatments, Dr K Tan restudied my case and prescribed RELPAX to treat my migraine.

Later I went to a government hospital for an MRI of my brain under Dr K Tan's suggestions. The result was all right – nothing wrong with my brain. I took that x-ray in 1985.

I must do my part not to rely on RELPAX all the time. On days when the migraine attacks did not occur, I should not take RELPAX. That's the goal. He managed the treatments on my ability to fight with myself without RELPAX (S$10 each medicine). It is vital to self-manage it.

I like four kinds of fruits that are high in antioxidants: tomatoes, watermelons, apples, and cucumbers.

I also took more vegetables—those reported to have increased in antioxidants.

I like tomatoes best because they are easy to prepare, and I can eat them as they are after a thorough cleaning. My stiff right hand evolves after typing at the computer for more than half an hour. The doctor recommended self-management discipline. Hence, after half an hour of typing credit proposals or reading relationship managers' credit proposals, I would take a rest.

What and how does a migraine-like?

I developed fright that affected my quality of life because migraine occurred daily. I had to take RELPAX daily (40mg max). It was a potent medicine. RELPAX is a brand name, and the generic name is El triptan hydrobromide (RxList, 2018). The common side effects of RELPAX include the following:

Mild headache (not migraine)

Tingling/numbness

Nausea

Upset stomach (a few occasions that I had migraine attacks that led to diarrhoea, and after passing motions, it would be all right after five to ten minutes)

Stomach pain or cramps

Drowsiness

You must share with the doctor if you have serious side effects of RELPAX as follows:

Blue fingers/toes/nails

Cold hands and feet

Dosage for RELPAX

A single dose of 40mg or other dosage is effective for the acute treatment of migraine, and after taking RELPAX, you must wait two hours before taking another dose. But that did not occur to me.

I tried to keep psychological balance, serving as a second reminder for my family and career.

Over time the stress built into my activities, although I could work if the migraine attack were on the way because my right hand stiffened up. The symptoms were a crystal that I would take the RELPAX medicine to stop it.

Although I was aware of the side effects of RELPAX medicine, unfortunately, migraine occurred daily. After taking

RELPAX, the stiffness on my right hand, right side of the neck, right eye, and brain would disappear within five to ten minutes (Dr K Tan, 2014).

The patterns developed until I was very fearful and consulted Dr K Tan, a neurologist. Migraine attacks only the right side of my body – hand, neck, brain, eye, and head. If I did not take RELPAX promptly, then my right hand, neck, eye, and brain would be in pain (how). So far, in 36 years, I only vomited twice. After vomiting, the migraine would recede within 10–20 minutes.

The author respects the knowledge of neurologist Dr K Tan in healing migraine. Dr K Tan's advice carried loads of weight and value and care.

Over the long and painful situations when migraine attacks occurred, I began with Ponstan and Cafergot given by the bank's doctor in 1980. It was terrible for me because it made my migraine worse. By then, I was already suffering from migraine. It was a daily painful experience. However, I continued to work after taking one each of Ponstan and Cafergot. It stopped the migraine within 15–20 minutes. They are painkillers, and they are potent medicines.

Dr K Tan continued to prescribe RELPAX (film-coated tablets, 40mg) from a private hospital neurologist to replace Ponstan and Cafergot to stop the migraine attacks because I loved my career in banking and finance. I suffered 36 years of migraine, since 1 February 1978 until Dr K Tan healed me on 1 March 2014.

I am fearful of migraine medicines because of the side effects. But I dealt with migraine under pain management and monitoring schedules and managed the stress of my banking-and-finance career. It was challenging because the Singapore Central Bank's Institute of Banking and Finance asked that

I impart my banking and finance knowledge and skills to division heads, SVPs, VPs, AVPs, managers, and specialists. That professional career was my first love.

Types of Migraine

A single dose of 20mg or 40 mg or other dosage is effective for the acute treatment of migraine, and after taking Relpax, you must wait 2 hours before taking another dose. Knowing the overdosage of REPLAX is the responsibility of acknowledge the side effect (negative) of REPLAX for patients' agreeing on their negatives and risk of overdosing the REPLAX. That helped the author overcoming the fear factors, and psychological balance of worries!

The author was meticulous on migraine medicines, and no overdose is the author's principle.

I tried to keep psychological balance, serving as a second reminder for my family and career. Over time the stress built into my activities, although I could work if the migraine attack were on the way because my right hand stiffened up. The symptoms were a crystal that I would take the RELPAX medicine to stop it from getting worse from my experiences that might lead to right neck, then right eye like needle poking may commerce. My diary recorded all these occurrences.

, But I was aware of the side effects of RELPAX medicine. Unfortunately, my migraine headaches occur daily. After taking the RELPAX, the stiff right hand, right-neck, right eye, and forehead would disappear within five to ten minutes. In the worst-case scenarios, it would affect my work. My diary record served as my reminders because the side effects of overdoes might occur.

That was the first line of defence for a healthy body.

From 1988 to March 2002, the Singapore Central Bank's Institute of Banking and Finance (IBF) requested me to be its qualified trainer and part-time lecturer to its collaboration with a UK university's MBA programmes. It also collaborated with Monash University for the Bachelor of Business (Banking and Finance) degree programmes. IBF requested me for helping under the instruction of the Singapore Central Bank (also known as the MAS). I was trying to give excuses not to help them. The Singapore Central Bank's IBF approached my bank's top management for approval that led to me in the situation that I could not reject it. The bank employing me approved it as a contribution to Singapore to be one of the global inancial centres because the bank is one of IBF's council members.

As regards to RELPAX medicine in April 2002 the patterns developed until I was very fearful and consulted Dr K Tan, a neurologist at a government hospital's NNI Clinic. Migraine headaches attack the only right side of my hand, neck, forehead, and eye. Migraine can be developed either from the left or right side of the patient's body. If I did not take the RELPAX promptly, then my right hand, neck, eye and forehead would be painful once it occurred. So far, for thirty-six years, I only vomited twice. After vomiting, the migraine would reduce within ten to twenty minutes. This is one of the possible patterns that developed for 36 years.

I had to keep a calm manner at work because I had mastered my Corporate Banking Head's work managing it in a foreign bank from 1997 to 1999., before I was approached by a mid- size government bank in December 1999 as a group head managing SME lending and Structured Trade Finance Group under Corporate Banking Division.

That was the only reason I must read loads of corporate banking knowledge, including syndications of loans and aircraft financing and structuring commodity financings. I am very conversant with legal documentation owing to the bank I worked for in the career that I loved. We must be familiar with legal documents and structures and clauses, apart from the deal's pricing.

Migraine

Migraine refers to a group of primary headache disorders marked by recurrent unilateral headache episodes. The doctor prescribed medicines for migraine, moderate headaches to severe pulsating pain, and it can go with nausea and increased sensitivity to light. However, I did not have such a symptom. I will share the patterns of my severe migraine in the following few chapters. I was fearful of migraine medicine overdose, it is harmful, and thus, it was out of the question for me.

I managed bank-lending businesses, from SME trade finance to corporate banking lending and projects. The migraine attacks occurred from my right hand (it stiffens), then right side of the neck and right eye, in a similar recurring pattern. I would have to take painkillers, such as Pons tan and Cafe got in the earlier days.

It can, unfortunately, develop into an unhealthy daily attack pattern. After March 2002, a friend asked me to visit a government hospital and see the neurologist Dr K Tan. Per the recommendation of a private hospital's doctor, I had changed to taking RELPAX for migraine, and Dr K Tan did not object to it after I consulted him, a neurologist from April 2002 until he healed on 1 March 2014.

What medicines help relieve migraine pain?

For mild and moderate migraine, doctors may prescribe over-the-counter medicines, such as Panadol or aspirin, to help relieve migraine (Giffin, N J et al., 2016; Bullock, 2020). However, by 1980, my migraine attacks were becoming severe, and the bank's doctors prescribed Pons tan and Cafe got. I have tried a few types of migraine medicines over the last 36 years until a friend referred me to a government hospital's neurologist, Dr K Tan, in April 2002 at NNI Clinic. The following drugs were prescribed at the beginning of my migraine attacks in 1978–1980:

> Aspirins
> Acetaminophen
> Acetaminophen, a combination of aspirins and caffeine
> Pons tan and Cafe got
> RELPAX

Summary of RELPAX

If the pain does not go away, more potent pain medicines may help. Thus, consult a doctor for use and if necessary, only for a brief period. The negative side effect is habit-forming (drug addiction), which is harmful to people who suffer from migraine. I was cautious of migraine medicines when my migraine attacks were so frequent and a common daily occurrence (Dr P Tang from 1988 to 1997 to whom I consulted).

A person can suffer from migraine once a year, but most patients may have suffered as often as daily (Saper and Magee, 1981).

I was sensitive to crowds. When I was in pre-university, I could not go to the cinema for a show because of lack of fresh air. Often, after the show, I would feel a heavy head. I suffered from migraine for 36 years, from 1 February 1978 to 1 March 2014.

Research revealed that most people who suffer from migraine are white-collar executives, and most of them are from blue-collar backgrounds.

The U.S. research showed that migraines might have a family background (Burch et al. 2018). Chronic migraine sufferers are women in the U.S., having 85% of sufferers being women, about 23 million women (Saper, MD, and Magee MD, 1981).

Usually, they would leave it to the doctor for treatments. It is a mistake! And attitudes or behaviour are that "I am not a doctor." Thus, I will let doctors treat me."

Most of them think that it is an extraordinarily prevalent neurological disease (Saper, 2018). The common tendency is to leave it to the doctor for treatments. The estimated number of people who suffer from migraine is about 39 million in the United States and one billion worldwide (Saper MD, 2018). In 1978, more than 30 million people suffered the incapacitating agony of recurring head pain in the United States (Saper and Magee, 1981).

Everything has its reasons in existence that are like migraines occurring in a person like me, which was because the workloads and the foreign exchange contracts for US dollars that the messengers must deliver timely to Treasury Division for import trade finance transactions that contracted and accepted by borrowing clients. The position must be covered for the day for all foreign exchange contracts (1978, a mid-size American bank).

That relates to pains or headaches in the forehead (either from the left or right side of the forehead) and it may be complex. However, those who suffer from it should consult a doctor, a specialist in migraine or pain management. The reasons may relate to stressful work or sitting in front of the computer to undertake work assignments for more than one to two hours, and that is because the sitting posture was incorrect.

I have suffered severe migraine attacks for 36 years since 1 February 1978 until 1 March 2014. In my case, it could be brought about by internal and external factors.

The internal factors included internal psychological issues such as messengers did not available to deliver the contracts timely to the Treasury Division and the human resources manager knew about it because I communicated with him that added press unnecessary on my work.

In short, it affected the quality of my life, facing recurring migraine pains daily because of the working environment in the bank that I worked for as head of the import trade finance department from 1975 to 1980.

The psychological reasons might have triggered my migraine attacks because of fears of stress! The overloaded work and assignments (projects) contributed by the messenger's delivery of foreign exchange contracts timely to the Treasury Division in the bank might be the reason! The human resources manager had meeting with all messengers in the bank, trying to resolve the issues with key performance indicators (KPIs) and specific duty.

What quality of life do I want to have? The migraine attacks affected the quality of my life, and the pain created fear in me. The side effects of migraine medicines are harmful and may create a vicious cycle of recurring pain at a fixed time, say, when

I wake up in the morning. Then I would take medicines to stop the pains from developing.

The antioxidant combination was effective in reducing the frequency and the severity of migraine attacks. Three months before the study, the study group suffered from migraine attacks at an average of 44.4 days per patient. (Goschorska et al, 2020)

A neurologist explains food triggers in children and how to conduct an elimination diet safely and effectively (Saper and Magee, 1981) that I must observe as pain management.

Migraine is a complex disorder with recurrent episodes of headache (Ashkenazi, A et al, 2007).

Common migraine risk factors include the following:

Family history
Medicines
Overdosage (may cause side effects)

Conclusion

If patients take RELPAX, they must avoid overdosage. The side effects may narrow blood vessels – a negative impact itself. To protect themselves, patients must record, like keep in a diary, their intake of RELPAX. It would be best to describe on record the migraine attack for patient safety and controlled management. At least the patients would know what is going on.

The migraine headache attack should be at the patients' figure tips (Giffin NJ et al.,2016) and that includes family history! The migraine headache sufferer's painful suffering should be recorded in a diary for references that is related to pain management, and I consulted Dr K Tan for control practices as a crystal record to prevent overdosage. It collaborated fine with me as a record to avoid overdosage that triggers side effect.

The author suggests that readers who experience migraine must keep a diary to record the occurrence of those migraine attacks. The author shares his experiences of migraine attacks in this book of nine chapters. When he finally recovered from migraine, the quality of his life improved, and he could concentrate on his works. Life would never be the same again. No fear factors would create fearfulness in his working life!

The author wanted healing and freedom from migraine. He viewed overdosage as a severe problem.

Even though the banking and finance job is my first love of my career, it did not stress me because I enjoyed the task and assignments. The problems that I had was at the mid-size American bank's messengers' delivery services were not acceptable to whom I discussed with the human resources manager for a solution, and it included key performance indicators that the Union agreed upon. That had been solved happily among all messengers involved in the bank.

My love in banking and finance and being Head of Corporate Banking Division in a foreign bank was my goal at the start that had never deviated from my goal. I always planned my works ahead of time and with consultation of other departments involved in acceptance of the changes, if any. That was to have a good working relationship among colleagues in other department or Division.

It concludes that the banking and finance career and assignments are my love for my job, and I enjoyed them so much! That was the expectation. I, the author, expected with an inclination to my professional works or assignments or projects.

I had endless energy for my professional career because of my first love of and passion of my banking and finance. The ultimate goal was to heal my migraines.

Chapter 2

My Migraine Journey Began
on 1 February 1978

I started recording in my diaries my migraine attacks (Appendix 1) on 2 January 1978, intending to find a cure. It was never an easy task to achieve. I suffered for 36 years, from 1 February 1978 to 1 March 2014 when Dr K Tan in the NNI Clinic healed me.

The first medicines I took were aspirin and Panadol.

The mid-size American bank's workloads were too heavy. It was because the short-handed situation. I was hoping it would improve after discussion with the human resources manager on this situation, especially the messengers were not always around to deliver foreign exchange contracts to Treasury Division that the clients had contracted, they were mainly in US dollar transactions.

I was so short of rest, and the overloaded work led to the stiffness of my right hand, occasional stiffness of the right side of the neck, pains in the right eye as if poked by a sharp needle, and migraine pains on the right side of the forehead. But Aspirin and Panadol were not working for me.

In 1980, the bank doctor changed the medicines to Pons tan and Cafe got. My migraine journey turned into a nightmare. They were addictive medicines; Pons tan and Cafe got are painkillers for migraine that almost destroyed my life. And the frequency of the migraine attacks were every other days. Later I left the mid-size American bank to protect myself from falling deeper into migraine problems.

After joining a local bank for less than a year, a prominent American bank offered me a position in marketing financial services to financial institutions (banks) as an assistant manager dealing with travellers' cheques, which were extremely popular those days. But this American bank's culture was not in the belief of teamwork for a few individuals, and it was clear that cooperation was missing. It made marketing travellers' cheques difficult to process in Japanese banks and other foreign banks too.

Shortly after this mistake, another prominent American bank employed me. I joined as an assistant manager, head of import trade finance department in trade finance operations division on 1 August 1983, and it was challenging for me. I was very experienced in import and export trade finance that I needed to manage about 12 staff, including a supervisor with proper experience and dependable performances. I have contacts with most of them today.

The American bank's doctor was helpful, and the doctor continued to prescribe Pons tan and Cafe got. But I worried about the side effects. I vomited twice in 36 years of migraine attacks. Before the bank sent me to Hong Kong for the Asia Pacific area's operations development management programme, the bank's seniors decided, selected, and assigned me as the coordinator for its commercial and retail loan system (CARLS) project. (I understood many people were aiming for it!) During this period, I had to work late, sometimes up to 2:00am. That worsened my migraine attacks and its frequency. I was cautious about the side effects.

Accordingly, the stresses level jumped up because I was still responsible for my import trade finance department. Apart from my responsibility shot-up, the volume also increased. I got my supervisor check all transactions and activities with the agreement of my VP boss. He told me, "It is all right, but I am holding you responsible!"

I would verify by the end of the day after all the important meetings for the CARLS project were over. Of course, I got my division head vice president to approve my arrangement.

These periods lasted for a couple of months until the CARLS project went live on 6 September 198. After the CARLS project was completed, we signed off with senior management. The chief credit officer (VP) wanted my signature on the documents. After the CARLS project went live on the scheduled date, the bank selected me to attend the Asia Pacific area's operations development management programme in Hong Kong. It was from 5 September 1985 to 6 December 1985.

It was a three-month programme for the Asia Pacific branches of the American bank. I met friendly and helpful managers from the Asia Pacific area. Some of them are excellent in English, while some are not so good. The Taiwanese and Japanese asked me for help. I had to manage my fee-based project proposal to be implemented in the Singapore office. I had to stay in Hong Kong for close to three months, from 5 September to 6 December 1985. My family joined me towards the end of the ODM programme.

While in Hong Kong, I visited the bank's doctor in Singapore on my concern and fear of migraine attacks, and the doctor was kind. I had to be in Hong Kong for three months. Thus, he prescribed three months' worth of migraine medicines to solve the concern.

Every morning all participants must be at the classroom at 9:00am. sharp. The senior executives were always punctual in starting the programme. All participants must complete the project assignments of their choice for assessments on the area of their interests and give them for examinations. At their requests, I did help a lot of Japanese and Taiwanese colleagues to correct their mistakes.

Things moved fast, and pressure simultaneously moved in the exact directions! My migraine attacks did not improve. It did not happen every day but on alternate days. When the other branches' participants asked me to help, we had to work as a team. I stayed at Elizabeth Apartment at Causeway Bay, facing the sea views even though the three-room apartment was small if I were to compare Taiwan and Japan.

However, the participants were helpful to one another.

One of the programme's uniqueness was that every participant would have to do a presentation relating to their projects. An untold feature was that the participants had to implement the tasks on their return to their branches. Thus, the assessments were strict, challenging, and business-driven for fee-based and interest incomes. Thank goodness, unlike in Singapore, my migraine attacks were not occurring daily for the three months.

The food streets in Causeway Bay had lots of attractive foods that made us aware of adapting cultures we learned from the programme. I usually do not eat beef, but the beef noodles offered was delicious. I began to take beef noodles on return to Singapore with my mother, wife, and two sons.

My project was expanding the fee-based income based on a structured finance that has risk, like back-to-back letters of credit structure that earned interest and fee incomes., suggesting widening the income-based on fee-income and interest-income taking credit and performance risk. The bank has an international network with excellent multi-national company clients with structured finance demands.

On completing the programme, my wife, two sons, and mother joined me in Hong Kong for a week before leaving on 6 December 1985. Yes, the migraine did not improve as expected to be all right! I continued to take the migraine attack medicines, Pons tan and Cafe got. But I was so careful not to overdose. Thank God's blessings! On returning to Singapore, the bank transferred me to the service products group of the corporate banking division to inject structured back-to-back L/C products having both credit and performance risks. That was the first time I managed structured trade finance facilities as service products in corporate banking division.

My project is on how can the bank's branch in Singapore increase fee-based income without additional risks on structured trade finance products and services in which the bank must know the clients' performance and credit risks.

The method is to increase fee-based income and interest income for structured trade finance products to manage the project, and the budget was US$5 million fee-based income for the coming year, 1985/86. I introduced the structuring of back-to-back letters of credit and forfaiting as products under service products that involved credit and performance risk considerations. We did complete the back-to-back structure for a large American diesel engine manufacturer on the confirmed L/C on a back-to-back basis. The buyer was a Thai company, and payment was on a 720-day L/C. I discussed this with the client's finance manager. He was promoted to CFO and transferred to New York HQs after the transaction was completed smoothly with closed monitoring as a structured finance. My bank approved the back-to-back L/C for the tenor of 720 days with pricing on L/C confirmation agreed and interest rate accepted for the entire 720 days financing period. The deal and structure became the bank's innovative product and forfaiting products.

The first deal was a back-to-back letter of credit structure on bus chassis for Thailand importer, of which the letters of credit was a tenor with 720 days (two years). Still, it must be on the confirmed letter of credit for the bank in Thailand to enjoy preferential fees and interest rates for its client, the importer.

The Singapore branch had the limit to take a two-year risk and approved a letter of credit. The amount of the deal was bus chassis assembly in Hungary's capital. The American bank that I worked with could take this structured deal to confirm the L/C for 720 days with a fee and interest rate agreeable for the Thai party. The value was US$5 million. The yield was reasonable, while the credit and performance risks were within prudential risk management of the American bank employing me. When I returned to Singapore after area office's operations management development programme, I increased the fee-based income under the service products group of the corporate banking division.

My migraine attacks came daily, and I recorded the level of migraine attack and position, for example, at the right side of the neck (RN-L5; 9:50am; RN = right side of the neck, L5 = the level of pains in a migraine attacks as shown in Appendix 1.

Therefore, I took one piece each of Pons tan and Cafe got to stop it and continued performing my duty as if nothing had happened. I was watchful of overdose. It lingered for five to ten minutes if I took it in the correct pain level. The recording method started in 1980 when the first bank's doctor changed my Panadol or Aspirin to Pons tan and Cafe got. From that day onwards, I was dependent on Pons tan and Cafe got because the vicious cycle occurred in the morning, on my waking time to send my second son to school and go to work. The migraine attacks were daily, and I needed migraine medicines to heal or stop the pains. But I worried about the side effects. It was captured and recorded in my diary.

As long as I could continue working with daily banking activities of meeting clients to structure trade finance under back-to-back letters of credit and asset-back financing using commodities as collateral supported by performance and credit risk evaluation, for example rubber as structured commodities financing for a long-established Singapore borrower in the rubber commodities business with Indonesia.

The service products group was able to meet the budget because the bank is a premium bank in the USA.

The forfaiting product is a structured and without recourse financing to the exporter of a commodity project. The tenor that forfaiting bank added its without recourse commitment for the entire financing period. The common one is 180 days commodities project financing. And for other project that may require three years without recourse to the exporter of the project financing. It needs a forfaiting bank to take the credit risks and get a forfaiting bank to take the risks with the fee and interest on without recourse financing. The financing is normally on financing large trade and commodities project financings for at least 180 days to the whole project financing of a maximum of 3 years that is common in the markets. That was in 1986 after I returned from Hong Kong's ODM programme.

I traced back in 1980 when the doctor changed the medicines to Pons tan and Cafe got. I began to record the frequency and occurrence of the migraine attacks. That was necessary because I did not want to depend on drugs, an unwelcome vicious cycle. So, I read books on fruits with high antioxidant levels, and I would consume tomatoes, watermelons, apples, and cucumbers as the books recommended. I ate the four types of fruits every day to ensure I had supply of the necessary and needed elements of vitamin C and antioxidants to reduce or prevent dependency or addiction, the side effect, to Pons tan and Cafe got.

By now, I had assumed my new role in the service products group and duty in the corporate banking division. For my health, I wanted to reduce the occurrence or frequency of the migraine attacks wherever possible. In June 1988, the bank promoted me to second VP for an excellent performance in the service products group, generating fee-based and interest income meeting the budget.

In August 1988, a prominent local bank headhunted me to be an AVP of marketing and customer service of trade finance. The bank promoted me to VP before the bank transferred me to be a team head of the commercial loans division, and the EVP knew that I was from the prominent American bank, where he also used to be a VP there. The transfer was in June 1990.

As a team head, I had eight relationship managers reporting to me. My credit analysis training was with a project at the American bank's area office in Hong Kong as part of the operations management development programme. I executed it in the Singapore head office in the service products group of the corporate banking division.

In the large local bank, I used my contacts to build the base for getting dependable SME clients. The bank had also set up an Indian desk to promote Indian businesses on fully-secured grounds according to the MAS standards. While it was so difficult to deal with Indian clients, the credit facilities must be on a secured basis. Again, the migraine attack was unkind to me. I managed my migraine attack on risk factor considerations, while fear factors were for my health management.

In 1992, the local bank selected me to lead the reengineering of the credit management programme using technology to help the credit appraisal and assessment process. We took about four months to complete the credit management project. Of course, in managing the project, there were agreements and differences in opinions. But after discussion, the members did not have any objections but agreed with conditions as criteria. The deal must agree with the requirements. We worked extra hours to meet our goals and aims.

On completion of the project, the management transferred me to head corporate banking, of which my responsibility was taking care of large deals and clients. Syndications of loans on aircraft financings and structuring of commodities financings and ship financings were also under my obligations.

As the business borrowing was extensive for corporate banking division. The structuring method was critical success factors because of larger amount of financing involved such as syndications of loans on aircraft financings, and ship financings. I also did structured commodities financings, assessing the performance risk that I needed to know the clients' operations in crystal.

Even though I had migraine attacks every morning, I had to manage it well not to lose any deal, especially syndications of loan financing involving billions of US dollars of projects.

The vicious cycle became normal more than abnormal. My migraine attacks recurred even more, and I wanted to challenge the repeating aggressive situation. Although I was fearful and the job was stressful, I managed and planned my work, and Pons tan and Cafe got became my companions.

No, I would not accept migraine attacks, and I would manage migraine attack and side effect risks.

I would try to be more relaxed in upgrading in terms of financing knowledge needed to buy the relevant books for my future career development and family future as a protection measure is the first priority without compromises on my migraines. My goal is to heal by neurologist doctor eventually.

But I never admitted defeat and fought migraine attacks finding migraine specialists and experts at the private hospitals.

Of course, I paid all fees myself for obvious reasons. I would not give up and believed that a neurologist would heal me one day, following a high-antioxidant fruit diet discussed in chapters 1 and 2.

A neurologist was consulted for treatments and advice to heal my severe migraine. That was the only goal of this book, for me to share my experience in the journey of combating migraine attacks. Readers can read the research study and story of an Australian migraine patient, Hanna (Bullock, 2020).

The classifications migraine are according to the International Headache Society (Giffin, N J et al., 2016). I was sensitive to crowded places, and I would avoid all the crowded places that possibly triggered my migraine.

Sometime in February 1997, a foreign bank headhunted me to be its head of corporate banking doing syndicated loans in aircraft financings and ship financings in addition to structuring commodities financings. It was because the bank's senior staff did not understand transferable loans facilities, amongst others. I talked with my friend, and he introduced me to his bank as a group head in SME and structured trade finance in the corporate banking division. That was November 1999, before the MAS encouraged the merger of banks during the Asia financial crisis period.

The bank offered me a position, as group head of SME and structured trade finance in the corporate banking division. I did a few structured trade finance deals and SME loans. However, my migraine did not stop. The bank's doctor also prescribed Pons tan and Cafe got.

Hence, I was very discipline to put curing my migraines a first priority as a control measure management while trying to relax in my love banking career.

In 2001, the MAS encouraged local banks to merge as large banks.

On about 1 June 2001, the merger was a success. However, the frequency of my migraine attacks continued to become an issue to me. The stiffness and pain on my right hand became a daily event. I could not type for five minutes at the computer.

Because it was a concern for me, I discussed with my wife that I might have to resign from the banking career I love. We set up an asset management firm in April 2002. A friend convinced me to visit Dr K Tan, a neurologist, a doctor for migraine, in a government hospital. Before that, I was under a private hospital's pain management doctor. He suggested I have four days of hospitalisation to get out the dependency on Pons tan and Cafe got. However, it was not successful. So my friend recommended that I consult Dr K Tan, a government hospital's neurologist, in NNI Clinic.

Conclusion

Pons tan and Cafe got may have triggered the addiction problems. I suffered from unexpected, unwelcome, vicious, and repeating migraine attacks. That nightmare is a painful suffering. It also created an adverse effect, a fearful factor amongst other risk factors. But I was confident that Dr K Tan would finally heal me.

That was a torturous life. It's negativity and fearsome factors could destroy an individual's confidence. On the other hand, it may be an opportunity to train and challenge an individual to overcome illness and difficulties.

I was inclined to take four kinds of fruits that are rich in antioxidants. It was better to have more fruits than to overdose on RELPAX. As explained in this chapter, I had never expected to suffer from migraine attacks.

Given my discipline in my work in the field of banking and finance, I firmly believe that I should not have migraine attacks, so I tried to check the reasons for my migraine.

Chapter 3

Doctor Requested Me To Stay In The Hospital For Four Days On Treatments To Reduce Dependency On Pons Tan And Cafe Got

After I resigned from the bank, I was under a private hospital's pain management doctor because my migraine attacks were so severe it results to pains in my right hand. The doctor suggested I have four days of hospitalisation to end the dependency on Pons tan and Cafe got. I accepted the hospitalisation for one goal: not to depend on Pons tan and Cafe got. The procedure to get rid of the addiction to or eliminate reliance on Pons tan and Cafe got needed four days of hospitalisation. And the cost was expensive, but I did not have a choice.

I could not type my credit proposal(s) for five minutes, and I could not lift my right hand, and the migraine attacks made me repeatedly consider my safety and family's. Before I decided on resigning from a banking career with a position of a VP(H), group head, which I loved, I discussed it with my wife.

A friend recommended that I must seek treatment and help from a neurologist for my migraine attacks at a government hospital. My friend led me to this good decision on March 2002.

My wife and I set up an asset management firm with two directors to manage the investment activities and engagements to preserve our savings and assets of 28 years.

However, it was not successful. So my friend recommended that I consult Dr K Tan, a neurologist at a government hospital.

The private pain management doctor changed my migraine attack's medicines to Pfizer's RELPAX (film-coated tablets, 20mg or 40mg). In migraine attacks, I experience stiffness of my right hand, neck, and eye.

Dr K Tan is committed to helping his patients recover from migraine. I cannot afford to pay for the private doctor's consultation, and cutting off from relying on Pons tan and Cafe got failed. It was time to change to a government hospital neurologist, and having a pioneer status, I was entitled to subsidies. My friend's suggestion was good.

I arranged for Dr K Tan to treat me with a 95% level of confidence. Dr K Tan is a neurologist for migraine at NNI Clinic at the government hospital. The journey began around April 2002, and I was impressed by Dr K Tan's knowledge in the neurological field. On the first visit for consultations, he examined me with an MRI scan to find my brain was all right. I told him I came to the hospital for an x-ray for my brain in 1985, and it was all right, nothing wrong with my brain.

After consultation, Dr K Tan told me to continue for few months on my migraine, and he will see me every three months. The day is always on Wednesday because Dr K Tan must visit the ward in the hospital in the morning and other days. I became confident, although RELPAX is expensive ($10 apiece).

My friend recommended to me to read up on a few antioxidants to understand the benefits of fruits and vegetables high Vitamin C and that it may help reduce the frequency of migraine attacks. I started reading books on fruits that are high in antioxidants. There are a few I like, such as (1) tomatoes, (2) watermelons, (3) apples, and (4) cucumbers. So reading books on antioxidants were essential to me to reduce the frequency of migraine attacks. I apply the method of thinking outside of the box for a solution in terms of my migraine illness. The goal is to read antioxidant fruits research study to find remedy besides relying on migraine medicines such as Pons tan Cafe got and REPLAX.

I also know that there are specific foods I must not take or avoid. I cannot have cheeses and cheesecakes for sure. I cannot have alcoholic drinks, like red wine or beer, because it may trigger migraine attacks. I am thankful to my friend, and I also consulted Dr K Tan and discussed the progress of my migraine attacks. Dr K Tan is a soft-spoken and kind-hearted neurologist, whom I respect.

Dr K Tan was aware of the high price of RELPAX. However, Dr K Tan believed that with it, I would eventually recover from my migraine. He knew discipline is essential in my daily activities, such as jogging 5–6km on alternate days to detoxify. With my commitment to jogging, Dr K Tan was happy with me. He knew I was careful on my fruits, vegetables, and food intake. He also knew I refused red wine or beer because alcohol would not suit me. I was committed to this discipline. Dr K Tan knew that my only goal was to heal my migraine, and I was also careful with the side effects of medicines for migraine.

Dr K Tan asked me to be calm with my plan to recover from my migraines and suggested not to force it as nature should take its causes of completing the task of investments. I must keep a calm behaviour to help myself end my migraine. I shared with him antioxidant fruits, vegetables, and foods, and he agreed to it.

My dear mum had always been concerned about my migraine and asked me to find time to relax to avoid having migraine attacks. I would share problems with her before her passing at 90 of age, on the first day of the Lunar New Year in 2017. When I woke up at 2:00am to look for migraine tablets, she knew that a migraine attack was coming.

I tried to remain calm at work, training bank managers at the Institute of Banking and Finance. I was well versed in the topics. I conducted training with case studies but kept the confidentiality of the cases. The real substance is assessing the credit risk or even performance risk in structured commodities financings. Running training sessions at the Institute of Banking and Finance for 16 years did not stress me. I enjoyed sharing knowledge and skills with participants from banks.

I always kept a piece of RELPAX with me, so if a migraine attack was on its way, I would take it to stop the attack.

I had to remain calm on the job at an asset management company, training bank talents in the Asia Pacific Region, including Malaysian and Indonesian banks and the central banks in these two countries. I could not rush it. All the bank managers and heads trusted me. The only stress was travelling to the venues in those countries to conduct the training programmes. It was necessary that I always have RELPAX with me for migraine.

The case study presentation of the group's findings was very appealing to participants. They learned more in taking part in the production, asking for justification and risk considerations.

The goal was to heal my migraine. I had been managing it, but I could not keep on depending on RELPAX because one of its risky side effects is thinning of blood vessels. I wanted to be healed entirely to be a healthy professional.

At this moment of writing, my banking and finance and asset management life is complex, but I am confident healing will also come in the end of my treatment by Dr K Tan, a neurologist.

My recovery was on 1 March 2014 amid my doctoral thesis research, aiming to compete with the Chartered Accountants from six public accounting firms supporting my research in July 2015. The overwhelming online responses was encouraging that I believe Singaporean Chartered Accountants are responsive for a good cause. I garnered 367 responses. Yet I could manage my migraine, encouraged by Dr K Tan.

On my recollection, I am thankful for Dr K Tan's effort to make things happen, healing my migraine before I finish my doctoral thesis writing. I am incredibly grateful to Dr K Tan who continued to check on me after recovery on 1 March 2014. Dr K Tan is a benevolent doctor who cured my severe migraine in 12 years, from April 2002 to 1 March 2014. Otherwise, I would not exist to share my challenging experience of migraine attacks with Singaporeans and those who suffer from migraine worldwide. After 43 years of migraine, the pains can kill me anytime. However, I read about fruits that are rich in antioxidants, vitamin C, and minerals. A friend recommended I take raw tomatoes that supply vitamin C, minerals, and the following (Togba, M et al., 2019):

Water: 95%
Calories: 18g
Protein: 0.9 grams
Carbs: 3.9 grams

Sugar: 2.6 grams

Fibre: 1.2 grams

Another friend recommended I take apples as it helps reduce tension and induce calmness. It is high in antioxidants and has vitamin C and minerals that are suitable for me, though it must be eaten and prepared like a vegetable (Togba M et al., 2019). We hear a common saying that "an apple a day keeps the doctor away." I read loads of articles and research papers on apples. Although I must take RELPAX, I also took an apple, and the other three types of fruits every day. My goal is to heal my migraine; to me it is an evil.

It also helped that I eat watermelon half an hour to 1 hour before meals. I developed this discipline strictly is to see positive results. I must also take cucumbers every day. This vegetable is high in antioxidants and has loads of vitamin C and minerals. I felt it in 2008 after consuming the four types of fruits from February 1978 with positive motivations.

The frequency of daily migraine attacks reduced at a slow pace until February 2014, while I was on my doctoral thesis research and writing my doctoral thesis supported by 367 samples provided by the Chartered Accountants online.

Conclusion

Migraine medicines were very unkind. The author took a lot of Pons tan and Cafe got as prescribed by the doctor. The author felt they were inappropriate because they were painkillers that led to the patient's reliance on them (Giffin, N J et al., 2016; Karsan N et al., 2018).

I did not know the medication was an addictive type of medicine. Even though I was careful, the vicious cycle of repeating migraine attacks developed to take centre stage. I was suffering like hell and fearful in my every waking hour, but I was determined and wanted to defeat those fearful feelings.

I hated to have developed dependency on RELPAX. Overdosage is harmful and risky.

That the patient of migraines may be dependent on the migraine medicines. It could be the risk factors of being overdosage.

Conclusion

In short, I had a phobia of migraine. Those were my fears, but I was confident that I would recover. Although the private hospital's pain management doctor tried to reduce my dependency on migraine medicines, the results were unsuccessful. My friend saw it and suggested I visit a government hospital's neurologist, DR K Tan. I was thankful to my friend that was an event under the way of recovery and healing. I only fearful on the migraine medicine. But I have no choice if I wanted to be healed support by subsidies for Pioneer Citizen and former National Service male, contributing to Singapore's defence.

Chapter 4

Antioxidant Fruits May Provide Vitamins C and K and Other Minerals to Reduce Severe Migraine

A private doctor recommended that I stay in a hospital to get over my dependence on Pons tan and Cafe got. It cost me few thousands of dollars without good results.

I went to a government hospital, NNI Clinic, to consult a neurologist, Dr K Tan, as recommended by my friend. I remember visiting Dr K Tan quarterly to review the treatments of my migraine. I was a cooperative patient because I wanted to be healed, and have a free of life transformation for the quality of life for contributing more to Singapore.

Dr K Tan was soft-spoken but thoughtful of the patient's fear, the recurrence of migraine and its risk factors. The migraine has been a daily occurrence since 1980. That made me feel I must heal it under Dr K Tan.

I remember I started in April 2002. I booked an appointment to visit Dr K Tan. While visiting Dr K Tan, I shared that I believed in antioxidant fruits, foods, and vegetables. I read loads of books on antioxidant fruits, and after my research, I consumed four kinds of fruits: (1) tomatoes, (2) watermelons, (3) cucumbers, and (4) apples. I would cook tomatoes, drink the soup in the morning, cut a tomato into two parts and use it to massage my right hand and forehead, each for one hour on 1 March 2014; the tension was because of my authoring my doctoral thesis research.

I would take uncooked cucumbers in the afternoon before lunch, and I must take one apple with pure tomato soup at night before dinner. At the time, I rubbed raw tomato on my right hand, and forehead too, if I feel stiffness.

Let me now review the four fruits as follows:

(1) Tomatoes

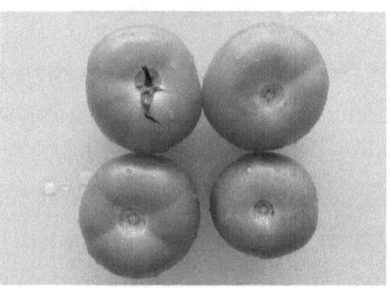

I had been eating this delicate fruit for 20 years under a pharmacist's recommendation, and I did not object to it. It has become my favourite fruit. I also cook soup without adding meat. Pure soup is better than anything! It calms my body and raise my body not to avoid my right-hand stiffened, with Vitamin C and Vitamin K's helps that may help to a certain extent for positive outcome, which was what I wanted.

Study revealed that tomatoes have a lot of relaxing elements. They are especially suitable for me. I used to rub tomatoes on my stiff right hand, and I never felt so relaxed. It was so relaxing, my hand felt like a child's, with not tension on my experience of rubbing with a tomato.

That day, on 1 March 2014 I used the other half tomato to rub my forehead for 1 hour with the same positive result – I had a relaxing forehead. That led me to refuse to take REPLEX. Tomatoes are one of the most consumed fruits globally (Jennings, MS, RD and Halial, APD, 2021). because they have so many vitamins, minerals, and bioactive compounds. Tomatoes are versatile fruits and are a rich source of vitamins, minerals, and antioxidants.

The picture of tomatoes is from 1978, and it shows the tomatoes I bought for my consumption because of my migraines. I have been cooking and eating them for 36 years, and I used tomatoes to rub them on my stiff right hand and tight forehead with positive results, meaning they became not stiffing on my right hand and forehead after rubbing for 1 hour each was relaxing!. Thanks to Dr K Tan's consultations (2013-2014).

(2) Watermelons

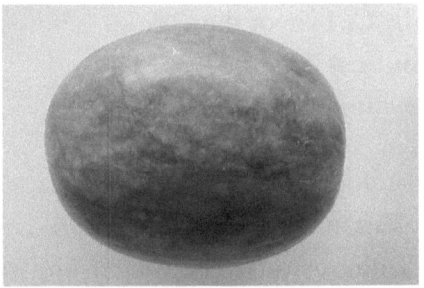

Watermelons have been over 4,000 years ago in Northeast Africa (Jennings, MS, RD and Halial, APD, updated on 8 November 2021). They become so common because it produces juices that help me a lot daily. I consume an 8 KG watermelon a week, and it makes my passing moments extremely easy in the morning. I think it as a detoxification process so welcoming to help my migraine.

Watermelons are high in antioxidants and vitamins A and C. It also has a variety of nutrients and potassium and magnesium. It's also relatively low in calories, containing just 46 per cup (152 grams) (5Trusted Source).

Watermelon is also a rich source of citrulline, an amino acid that may improve exercise performance (6Trusted Source).

It is sweet and juicy, making it a perfect treat to quench your thirst during the summer heat.

Here are the nutritional values in a cup (152 grams) of raw, diced watermelons:

> **Calories:** 46g
> **Carbs:** 11.5 grams
> **Fibre:** 0.6 grams
> **Sugar:** 9.4 grams
> **Protein:** 0.9 grams
> **Fat:** 0.2 grams
> **Vitamin A:** 5% of the Daily Value (DV)
> **Vitamin C:** 14% of the DV
> **Potassium:** 4% of the DV
> **Magnesium:** 4% of the DV

Eating fruits, like watermelon, is a crucial way to keep the body healthy. Watermelon is a plant species that bears flowers that becomes fruits of different weight and several colours. The common one is red and juicy, and there is also a yellow variant. (Wikipedia, November 2021). I like watermelon very much, and I have been eating a large one (8kg) every week for 36 years since 1 February 1978. It also refers to packed with nutrients, including antioxidants and vitamins A and C. Leaves are alternate, simple lobed or palmately compound. It improved my motion discharge at ease every morning for year. It could increase the detoxification from my personal experience.

(3) Cucumbers

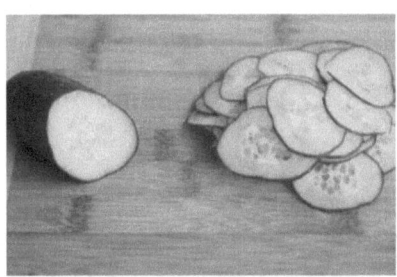

Cucumbers have excellent benefits: low in calories and high in many essential vitamins and minerals. (2Trusted Source).

An unpeeled raw 11 oz (300g) cucumber has the following (2Trusted Source):

> **Calories:** 45g
> **Total fat:** 0 grams
> **Carbs:** 11 grams
> **Protein:** 2 grams
> **Fibre:** 2 grams
> **Vitamin C:** 14% of the RDI
> **Vitamin K:** 62% of the RDI
> **Magnesium:** 10% of the RDI
> **Potassium:** 13% of the RDI
> **Manganese:** 12% of the RDI

Cucumbers (*Cucumis sativus* L.) belongs genus in family and is an easy fruit vegetable that is affordable (Jia and Wang, 2021). Cucumbers are vegetables, not fruits. They are about

96% water and may help you keep hydrated and meet your daily fluid need. It calms my nerves and stress at work and help prevent migraine attacks. I take it every other day.

Cucumbers have a lot of vitamin C and cause no harm to the body. Cucumbers also have vitamin K that help improve calcium absorption. These nutrients keep good bone health. Cucumbers also have vitamin D, an essential for bone health (Ware, 2019).

(4) Antioxidants of Apples

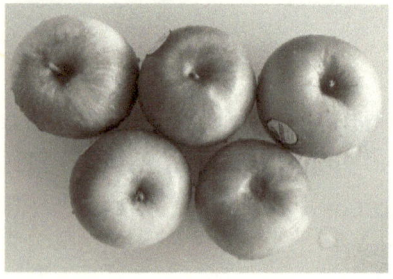

Researchers found that apples are significant sources of flavonoids in diets in the United States and in Europe (Boyer and Liu, 2003). In the United States, 22% of the phenolics consumed from fruits come from apples, making apples the most significant source. We have been hearing at a young age, "An apple a day keeps the doctor away." The author took an apple every day and likes it in different colours.

Boyer and Liu's research (2003) revealed that many cultures commonly enjoy apples, which are a good source of antioxidants. Because of this, I started taking apples to reduce my migraine. As researchers discover increased evidence to support the role of phytochemicals in decreasing the risk of chronic disease, some have hoped to find a magic bullet that prevents chronic illness.

I visited a government hospital as a first batch National Service male and commissioned an arm forces officer without the problem of migraines. The contributions were there, and it also trained us to be a fit person.

Keeping fit has become my personal belief for my health, safety, and family. Being a self-disciplined National Service male fitness is number one to my family, wife, two sons, me, my mum. My two sons are working in professional fields. My elder son is working in the banking and finance sector and is a Chartered Accountants.

He holds an SVP position in a large bank; likewise, his wife is a chartered accountant and SVP in another large private bank.

My second son, whom I respect, is a medical doctor holding a Masters of Medicine (Family) with an MBBS from the NUS. His wife is also a Masters of Medicine (Psychiatry) holder with an MBBS from the NUS, now working in a government hospital. They have a daughter (elder) and a son (younger) and kept to themselves, building their family. My granddaughter and grandson are loveable like that of my elder grandson from my elder son. He is well behaved.

I tend to relax when I play with my three grandchildren; seeing them playing in freedom means the growing environment is different nowadays. Readers can read my other book, My Mother's Love (Tan, 2021).

From April 2002 until today, 18 November 2021, it is more than 18 years, but I fully recovered on 1 March 2014 (about 12 years after Dr K Tan healing me).

But from 1978 until 2014, a total of 36 years, I suffered migraine attacks fearfully.

During consultations, Dr K Tan and I discussed my improvement in treatments, and he gives me pieces of advice; my confidence is raised to the direction of seeing myself medically all right. Healing and freedom from migraine is critical for my family and children and grandchildren.

I respect Dr K Tan's caring and kind heart. He patiently listens before deciding on what medicines to prescribe. That part of the consultation made me realise that patient listening will lead to a more correct diagnosis. At the beginning of consultation with him, I was already confident that Dr K Tan would lead me towards the healing of my migraine. But I must be patient. There was a good chance that he would heal me, seeing how he was committed to diagnosing intently. When he suggested a preventive migraine medicine of 300mg, I told him I would try it. I made a record in my diary, indicating the date and time. Dr K Tan's visiting appointment is always on Wednesdays, around 9:15am.

I had already tried the preventive medicines for three months in the next appointment, but it was not working for me. Therefore, I got Dr K Tan's assessment, and he decided to drop this preventive medicine, and it decided to review in the next three months. It was all right to meet my goal of healing my 43 years suffering from 1978 to 2021. But I recovered on 1 March 2014, 36 years.

So to be precise, from 1 February 1978 to 1 March 2014, it is 36 years of tortuous migraines.

Thank you, Dr K Tan and God's blessings my migraines that my migraine would heal in the near future. It was always on the right side of my hand (stiffness), right-neck (stiffness and pains), right-eye (like needle poking pains), and right- -forehead pains.

I saw Dr K Tan four times a year. He was also committed to help me with my goal: heal my migraines. I gained more confidence after each visit to Dr K Tan. I continued to take antioxidant fruits and vegetables as recommended by the books. The books' authors are pharmacists, and thus, they have a medical background.

My treatment by Dr K Tan from April 2002 up to today is already Nineteen years. But I gained my full recovery on 1 March 2014. I am now confident that it will not come back. Therefore, in the next consultation, I will discuss with Dr K Tan to keep my future appointment dates open for optimize the scarcity of resources.

That day I read my doctoral research and planned to meet with the CEO of Singapore Accountancy Commission (SAC), reporting to the Ministry of Finance. My right hand gave a signal of stiffness and right forehead tightness. I took a small tomato and cut it into two pieces. I started massaging my right hand for one hour. A miracle happened: My right hand was fully relaxing like a baby's hand, without stiffness.

I was happy. I did the same massaging to my forehead's tightness for one hour, and a similar feeling took place. It was a miracle to me, although I had been taking tomato soup for 6 years. I stopped taking RELPAX on 1 March 2014.

I recorded this event in my diary according to my ten grades stated in Appendix 1 (Chapter One; from grades 1 to 10).

My right hand's stiffness was at about level 5, while my forehead's tightness was at about level 4–5 after rubbing it with the other half tomato for one hour. My right side of my head was so relieved, like no tension (Giffin, N J et al., 2016). I continued to take the four fruits that are high in antioxidants as mentioned. I recorded in my diary my recovery from migraine without RELPAX! Thank you, Dr K Tan!

No RELPAX for me since 1 March 2014 gave me confidence. In 36 years of suffering, that was the first time, since 1 February 1978. When I met up with Dr K Tan in about April 2002 I thanked him sincerely for his benevolent and consideration in his medical treatments.

God's blessings from that day onwards with my commitment in taking tomatoes, cucumbers, and their soups. I also eat apples every day.

The evil migraines never came back.

Thank you, Dr K Tan, for the antioxidant fruits and vegetables that I took for 36 years after reading the antioxidant book's recommendations to the four types of fruits mentioned in the chapters.

On 1 March 2014, I stopped taking RELPAX migraine medicine and after taking antioxidant fruits and vegetables from 1 February 1978 to 1 March 2014.

I used the tomatoes to massage my stiff right hand and the heavy right side of my forehead (level 4 – Appendix 1). The stiffness disappeared after one hour of massaging. both my right-hand and right forehead on 1 March 2014.

Now, I understand what is the quality of life without migraines? I had been happy to help my father and mum on their business on spring sprouts. Dr K Tan knows my family backgrounds very much and wanted to heal me with no pressures. The pain management doctor at the private hospital changed my migraine medicines to RELPAX. Dr K Tan continued to prescribe RELPAX but was at a standby treatment until I fully developed confidence.

Since 1 March 2014, I have not taken RELPAX anymore, and it has been an achievement since 1 February 1978. But I did not take it because I needed to gain my confidence.

In my next visit to Dr K Tan, I want to discuss with him to keep my consultation dates for the future appointments open because I am confident with my health now. I hope the hospital can consider put me on a standby basis.

Thank you, Dr K Tan, for treating my severe migraine in April 2002.

Since I totally recovered from my migraines on 1 March 2014, I could contribute more to Singapore on asset management investments and continue my experience in banking and finance, authoring books on my experience of 28 years in corporate banking and structured trade finance and commodities financings.

Conclusion

Fruits that are rich in antioxidants are common, and they have no side effects. However, I shall not overeat but keep a healthy habit of eating fruits and vegetables to keep migraine at bay. Antioxidant fruits helped me reduce my dependency on Pons tan and Cafe got.

However, the unsuccessful four days of hospitalisation made things worse. The private hospital pain management doctor changed my medication to expensive RELPAX. I could not support myself financially on RELPAX. I requested a friend to recommend me take me to a government hospital for migraine treatments under its NNI Clinic. The reason is that I am a pioneer citizen who is eligible for subsidies.

Antioxidant fruits, such as tomatoes, watermelons, cucumber, and apples, would be more helpful to the author than RELPAX. I added with my exercise routine on alternate day at 5KM running (or jogging if I am tired that day. The exercise is paramount important for me since I was serving my Nation Service in arm forces as a commissioned Armed Forces Officer.

Chapter 5

Costly Illness and Risk and Fear Factors

Costly illness may be a serious concern. Treatments for migraine are not cheap.

Migraine (Rayne, K A et al., 2011; Blooed et al., 2012) is a costly illness, risky of overdoses, raising of fear factors that created adverse consequences, despite severe side effects!

The author was careful and was saved by the compassion and care of Dr K Tan, a neurologist at a government hospital's NNI Clinic. The author began counting the cost involved from 1 February 1978 until today.

1985 was an x-ray on my brain, but 1990 was an MRI on my brain at the government hospital. The record shown that my brain is all right.

Those were costly even with the government's subsidies for pioneer patients like me, the first batch of National Service Male, contributed to Singapore's defence.

The second contribution was in the banking and finance sector because Singapore Central Bank's Institute of Banking and Finance requested me to be a qualified trainer and part-time lecturer. They got my employing bank's top management approval that I could not reject. It was to ensure Singapore will be one of the global financial centres, ranking third or fourth position. I contributed to the banking and finance sector in a welcoming manner.

The syndications of loans involving aircraft financings and ship financings were under my care in the corporate banking division.

I started my banking and finance career on 1 February 1975 after being discharged from National Service obligations. My migraine was brought about by my job as head of import trade finance, which was short-handed, in 1978. Unfortunately, my migraine began to develop, and initially, the bank's doctor prescribed medicines like Aspirin and Panadol. In 1980, the frequency of migraine attacks did not decrease but rather increased.

By October 1980, a local bank invited me to join the bank's international banking division's import trade finance department. Even though my employment bank has medical benefits, I must visit the doctor for ordinary migraine. However, when I was referred for treatment to a neurologist in a private hospital, at Mt. Elizabeth Hospital's migraine clinic, I had to bear all costs myself. That cost a bomb on my bills. Therefore, I saved a lot of my income after CPF contributions under laws.

(Department or group, team will start with the alphabet in Capital. It is a rule - similar to our name. Please do not include this in the book.)

I did not see improvement, so I went back to the bank's panel of doctors for migraine medicines. But it did not work fine for me. I suffered loads of stress, although I love my job. There were billions of US dollars of financings for lending to large world-class companies with good business models.

The author shares three analyses to the readers, and they are as follows:

Life and healthcare
Migraine and costly illness
Migraine, risk and fear factors, and side effects
of RELPAX

Life and Healthcare

A person should live a healthy life so that the person can contribute to the country. positively.

The author did not know if there was any correlation with his birth's diarrhoea illness. The author should thank his dear mum with respect. Without her care, the author might not have survived. There was a challenge growing up with the author and helping the author's father and mum in their spring sprouts business.

The author's father had a lot of expectations from the author. The author's starting life was tough, but his endurance transformed him. That becomes his trademark of a person has high motivation in any assignments! He trained to be a tough person with a goal and two objectives (aims). Because of the dear mum and medical team's care, he survived under the extreme difficulty of growing up with diarrhoea at birth.

Life is the fact that the author must deal with.

The author now keeps his life with a guided procedure and sufficient exercise to have a healthy body and reads daily in two languages, keeping the brain cells active and can take more reading of acquiring knowledge.

Migraine and Costly Illness

Those who suffer from migraine (Giffin, N J et al., 2016; Karsan, N et al., 2018; Steiner, T J et al., 2018) will typically say it is a costly and torturous illness. Hence, those who suffer from it must constantly manage the illness with great care and always remain calm amidst undeniable work stress. Again, the author developed his motivation to have challenges. But I love my career in banking and finance.

And you, my readers, are learning from my sharing of daily migraine attacks. The author dealt with migraines for 36 years, from 1 February 1978 until 1 March 2014, and the author had fully recovered since.

Thanks to Dr K Tan, a knowledgeable neurologist. Apart from being a costly illness, the medical treatment for migraine is a painful process. Thus, you must set a goal to heal yourself under a government hospital.

Government hospitals have neurologists with subsidy and Medisave from CPF to lessen medical treatment costs. The author suffered from the cost and physical pains for 36 years. Without his dogged determination, he may not have made it to the pinnacle of life although it was a tough but happy journey for him, and his family and two sons and three grandchildren. God's blessings in me appear crystal, and healing the migraine is a gift for goal to have the quality of life!

The author suffered migraine since 1978, although he was all right in serving his National Service (NS) obligations (being the first batch of NS males born in 1949) as the migraine illness did not happen because the field training in military was at open air. But field training was under the hot sun Although the author was all right in the field, the author needed fresh air and must avoid crowded places. Those are the reasons I know even until today. Otherwise, I may not have recovered from migraine!

I experienced pre-university in 1968, and the Ministry of Education implemented the Junior Colleges Scheme in 1969.

Before serving National Service obligations, the author was in pre-university (now A levels).

I would not go to the cinema for shows because after a show, my head was heavy. From my observations, I needed to have fresh air. I also avoid crowded places, not allowing myself to have a heavy head. That could be the start of a migraine attack. The author tried to analyses it as a precaution.

After authoring his first two books—one title, but one in English and one in Mandarin (Dr Tan 2021)—the author wanted to share his migraine experience and tortuous sufferings with my readers. In this book, the author wanted to share with the people who suffer from migraine in Singapore, costing Singapore S$1.04 billion in 2018 (Ong et al. 2019). In the USA and world-wide migraine patients. Research showed in the United States of America there are 85% of women suffer from migraine – a total of 23 million. But world-wide, it is in the tune of one billion people, awaiting treatments and with the hope of recovery.

In his goal and two objectives (aims), the author tried to describe the situations of migraine in Singapore (, (Tan, 2021).

However, the author started his banking and finance career as a bilingual, speaking excellently in English and Mandarin. He suffered from migraine since 1978, and he was so happy that he recovered on 1 March 2014 healing by Dr K Tan, the neurologist.

Migraine, Risk and Fear Factors, and Side Effects of RELPAX

Patients of any illness need to consult doctors and take medicines as directed for treatments. We heard of overdoses and side effects of drugs. Patients must ask their doctors about the side effects of migraine medicines. For example, if a doctor prescribes Pons tan, Cafe got, RELPAX, or other drugs to reduce attacks or cure migraine, one of the side effects is the narrowing or thinning of blood vessels, which may be risky for patients with other illnesses. Further, for self-awareness and protection, patients must also ask their doctors what foods trigger migraines.

The author summarised below the common symptoms of migraine attacks (the Migraine Trust, 2021; Steiner, T J et al., 2018):

Pain on the right side of the head
Pain on the right eye
Stiffness on the right side of the neck
Stiffness of the right hand
Vision difficulties
Sensitivity to lights, sounds, and smells

The author had to take RELPAX daily (40mg max). RELPAX is a brand name, and the generic name is El triptan hydrobromide (Rayne KA et al., 2011; RxList, 2021). But the author did not want any prevention of migraine medicines.

The author must share with the doctor if he has serious side effects of RELPAX as follows:

blue fingers/toes/nails, or
cold hand and feet

Serious Side Effects

This list has examples of severe side effects that can occur with Relpax and Maxalt (when taken individually):

> Serious heart and blood pressure problems (attack)
> Problems with blood circulation, such as lack of blood flow to your nose, ears, fingers, or toes ("Imitrex: Side effects, dosage, how it works, and more")

Effectiveness of RELPAX

RELPAX can treat migraine with or without aura in adults. The drugs have no clinical studies, but studies found REPLAX to treat migraine with or without aura effectively.

Migraine and Fear

Fear and productivity are correlated. Presenteeism (present but low in productivity) and absenteeism (totally nonproductive) are two expected outcomes of fear, and they can be associated with risk factors. Worse can happen to fearful migraine patients.

No organisation can have sick employees. When employees are ill and not healthy, it affects their outputs or contributions, and the result may be harmful. Thus, wealth for any individual in the working class is essential.

The fear factors are common in migraine patients and any sick person for that matter, and it may lead to negative moods and situations, like overdose, amongst others. Hence, eat healthy and keep a healthy body.

The author used a grading system with the levels indicating when migraine attacks are on the way. This method would also prevent a patient from overdosing.

Study showed that fear factors are the pain when migraine headaches occur without the patients knowing, and it becomes a risk factor without taking the migraine medicines. It is because the patients may not have experience in the timing of migraine headache attacks. To buy the ability, the readers can refer to chapter 1's suggestion based on the level of grades records to guide you in chapter 1. The author managed the guided level of grades (Appendix 1) on the future migraine headaches. The author summarises below as a guide shown in chapter 1.

The Study of Mood and Migraine Relationship

A survey of more than 30,000 participants in a Canadian study showed that major depression, bipolar disorder, and social phobia were all at least twice as prevalent in migraine subjects. The findings were not in demographic and socioeconomic variables (Fanning et al., 2012; Belmonte C, et al., 1991).

The findings illustrating the relation between mood and depression were clear. The risks of and fear of depression and anxiety in migraine are not surprisingly related to headache burden. One study showed a linear relationship between headache frequency and the odds ratio of depression or anxiety (Kawata et al., 2011; Joel R. et al., 1981). Hence, the motivation factor is more important to stabilise the occurrence of migraine.

I constantly reminded myself not to overdose because the migraine medicine is potent, so I must manage it rigorously, without compromising for my personal protections. To me, health is also my priority, and it may have related to the level of stress.

What can you do to help manage your migraine?

Those occurrences of migraine attacks were my experiences from 1 February 1978 to 1 March 2014, 36 years of serve sufferings! However, the migraine attacks became a vicious cycle in the morning, and the patterns were healthy. They are harmful to the mood or psychology. *I used to tell myself I would conquer it and that I could not be my enemy.* I would check it and work happily at my banking and finance career. Thanks to Dr K Tan's treatments and consultations, on 1 March 2014, the day I defeated migraine and achieved freedom and a changed life.

My horizon opened for my patience, awaiting 36 years of fearful life if not because of my love of banking and finance career motivating me to get doctor to cure my migraines.

The most challenging part of my banking and finance career life was when the Singapore Central Bank's Institute of Banking and Finance appointed me as a qualified trainer and part-time lecturer. I am thankful to them.

Nowadays, I am careful about my daily activities, and exercises have become a regular discipline and habits that I cannot ignore. The author consumes fruits high in antioxidants, such tomatoes, watermelons, cucumbers, and apples, based on personal research. That is my way of preventing migraine and keeping myself healthy.

It was priceless to heal my migraines by Dr K Tan. The author considered his recovery from my migraine headache on 1 March 2014 because the treatments and healing medicines were so important. I always recorded in my diary that not overdosing is allowed.

My brain is crystal-clear without migraine. The author wanted to share his sufferings and experiences for 36 years with readers like you.

The author will consult Dr K Tan after his recovery on 1 March 2014, 8 years ago. Going forward, the author may ask Dr K Tan to keep it an open date as a stand-by of his protection in the coming consultation four months later, April 2022.

It was my reason for asking Dr K Tan to continue to give me treatments and consultations until the author gained his confidence with no occurrence of migraine headaches!

Overall, the author suffered loads of stress, internally and externally, from migraine attacks.

The author shares with readers a neurologist commitment to healing the author's migraine.

Conclusion

The author appreciates Dr K Tan's treatments, consultations, and knowledge in neurology. If my recollection is correct, I was with Dr K Tan for treatments in April or May 2002. After the first consultation, I reminded myself to heal my migraine attacks. The pains of migraine attack did not defeat me, but they gave me courage and the spirit to fight migraine. My conclusion had something to do with my book My Mother's Love (in English and Chinese, Dr Tan, 2021).

However, as of 1 March 2014, I no longer need to take RELPAX. Thank you, Dr K Tan, for your patience and knowledge. I requested Dr K Tan's permission to continue to consult me until such a time I am confident in dealing with my situations. Even though it may take years, I will not allow lapses to happen.

I have complete confidence in my neurologist Dr K Tan. I learned patience from him as it relates to migraine. We will proceed to the next chapter to determine the progresses on the treatments that healed me on 1 March 2014.

Chapter 6

The Neurologist Healing My Migraine

My Goal – A Thriving Career in Banking and Finance and a Happy Family

No one wants to suffer pains from migraine attacks. However, if you suffer from migraine, you, as readers, must learn from the author prevention of such migraine attacks, and find out the internal and external factors to know himself or herself better in a strategic management of migraines.

The author's first love is his banking and finance career supported by his health condition to cut his migraine headaches.

The author feels authoring the book contributes to Singapore and the world at large, sharing his experiences in the bumpy life journey, suffering from migraines from 1 February 1978. Readers may want to read the author's first two books on the challenges of his growing stages – in English or in Chinese. I succeeded in using my nine principles, offering a takeaway for you on asset and liability management model in the first two books (Dr Tan, 2021).

If you are a migraine patient, you must consult with and be under the treatments of a neurologist. That is crucial because they are trained specialists to treat and heal migraine brought about by work and incorrect sitting position in front of the computer. As advised by doctors, do not sit at the computer, to type or work, for more than half an hour.

One of the protective measures is to check with your doctor, the neurologist on overdoses of migraine medicines prescribed by the neurologist.

The bank's doctors are family doctors, and thus, they are not neurologist. The author is thankful for the patience and care Dr K Tan had, especially at this time.

The author first met Dr K Tan at NNI Clinic, and the author shared his migraine attacks since 1 February 1978. Under Dr K Tan's care, with his experience and knowledge, I began to see gradual improvement. His care and patient treatment impressed me. He detailed all consequences. Dr K Tan prescribed medicines for three months, and I visited him every three months.

Top management of the bank employing me approved Singapore Central Bank's request to appoint me as a qualified trainer and part-time lecturer for its Institute of Banking and Finance in 1988

Of course, I got my superior's (EVP) recommendations and top management's approval because the bank employing me was a council member in 1988. The rest are history.

Per the request of the Institute of Banking and Finance, my role as a trainer and mentor was to share my knowledge, skills, and experiences, through cases studies, with the participants.

Managing the Reengineering of Credit Management and Assessment Project

In 1989, the bank appointed me to be a coordinator (or leader) of the reengineering of the credit management project using technology to support the whole process according to the bank's credit policies.

Hence, I must organise it with the team for the project. The challenges were my migraine attacks that occurred daily, and I had to manage them carefully without hurting myself. In those days, the bank's panel of doctors prescribed me Pons tan and Cafe got.

After four months, we completed the reengineering of the credit management project. Then the management transferred me to corporate banking, responsible as a team head for highly valued clients. The author managed syndications of loans for an aircraft financing project for an essential client with manageable risk. The borrower requested the bank to inject US$5 million on the equity side apart from loans. On the other hand, the bank's part as the lender was the key. Therefore, I had to manage loans and equity investments responsible by the Corporate Investment Division.

The Open Sky's My Limit in My Banking-and-Finance Career

The author suffered from migraine, and it occurred daily. He was also concerned with overdosage, regardless of whatever situation.

Another financing project, such as ship financing, was a big challenge. However, the author chose an experienced relationship manager who could assess all documents apart from the structures and legal documentation. The author could still control his migraine, although the frequency of migraine attacks became daily, falling into a vicious life cycle. The author managed to prevent overdosage, recording in his diary.

Self-Disciple and Development of Health and Wealth (Savings and Investments) Regardless of Migraine Difficulties

No one can help my migraine attacks. Although the work was very stressful, I loved this kind of challenge and upgrading my knowledge to help the Institute of Banking and Finance (IBF) with its training programmes that approved by the IBF with case studies for practices. The People's Bank of China wanted Singapore Central Bank's help with the World Bank on credit risk management and case studies. From 1997 to 1999, the People's Bank of China asked the Singapore government and the World Bank for credit risk management and case studies programmes. It was twice a year – in March in Beijing and in September in Shanghai. The chairman of the People's Bank of China requested the author to conduct the training programmes using Putonghua and the World Bank's trainers supported the request. The author did, and they were so happy! The author had been managing his migraine attacks very well.

Managing my investments from my Savings suggested by my colleague in the large American bank

In 1985, the author started investing as advised by his colleague in a large American bank.

The author's colleague told him that he must learn how to protect his savings for investments. However, the author used Warren Buffett's value investing methods. The author bought many books on Buffet's strategies. However, managing migraine attacks was still the author's top priority.

The author learned from this colleague how to protect his savings. However, the author is a conservative person who was not taking higher risks. The author discovered investing as an education guided by his tertiary study. And the author would not compromise on his migraine attacks. The author had been disciplined in his health trying to heal his migraine by avoiding Pons tan and Cafe got. The side effects may eventually be harmful to him. The author managed his health for the sake of his family, his wife, two sons, and future grandchildren.

His first love is his professional career in banking and finance. The author could not foresee the future, but he hopes for the best to see he recovers one day. That would make him continue to contribute his knowledge to Singapore.

Confidence in Future Events and Endeavour

A healthy body is essential to the healing of the author's migraine. It will yield better-investing results and contribute more to Singapore intellectually. The author has produced two books, in English and in Chinese, titled *My Mother's Love* (Dr Tan, 2021).

COVID-19 caught everyone by surprise. No one can predict the future, but one's health should be in one's hands going forward.

The author has set the rule that he enjoys it with his grandchildren one day, using motivational method of playing and learning. No more learning by hard without the mentality of non-creative teaching.

Conclusion

Migraine is terrible, and it has put me in a difficult situation. Hence, I must recover from migraine. I did 5km jogs on alternate days. I want to contribute to Singapore in asset management investments, banking and finance, a red dot to an influencing red dot without migraines.

Migraine pulled me back for many years and forced me to protect myself from resigning from OCBC Bank.

I could not use my right hand to type credit proposals or work for more than five minutes. I decided to preserve my life and family, and I resigned on 31 March 2002. I wanted to change my life and be free of migraine in the next few years.

My plan should and must happen if I get back my confidence.

When would it happens? I did not know. But after consulting with Dr K Tan of NNI Clinic, a government hospital clinic, I have complete confidence to see that day coming into my life, and I will be relaxing with my three grandchildren.

The only time that I can relax is when I'm playing with my three grandchildren, and I want to see them growing up happily.

Chapter 7

Managing Stressful Working Life – Loving Your Career

The author read loads of books on antioxidants to gain knowledge and only took fruits that are suitable for him. It significantly helped reduce his migraine attacks.

By March 2002, the author faced difficulties at work, like typing credit proposals after getting the deals. It was a concern, and the author checked with his wife and discussed that he might have to resign because of this problem.

The author's second son had excellent A level results (scored As for all subjects). The author would support his second son's medical study. Not everybody has that kind of opportunity. The author had been saving for 28 years for this day.

Never Overdose and Risks

Overdoses of migraine medicines may be risks to a patient. Those were the side effects of migraine medicines. Hence, I recorded the occurrence of migraine and the medicines I took in my diary as a control management. I have no exception from 1 February 1978.

In a migraine attack, the pains are in the nerves of the brain (either side of the brain), and the brain is in pain. The author imagines that your blood vessels are in pain.

Imagine your migraine attack as a daily occurrence. The author must have been strong to create records and overcome the pain. Although the medications are costly, this situation may lead patients to overdosage. Then you lose your confidence. Then the problem falls into a vicious cycle. The author was at that stage of overdose. The severe migraine attacks destroyed his confidence.

Strong Belief in Self-management for Health and Wealth

It was because I suffered from migraine headache attacks underpinned by both internal and external factors.

One of internal factors was that my parents needed my help in their spring sprouts business. Every day I worked four to five hours helping my parents when I was young. In my young life, I was rushing to find the time to study, and I must complete it no matter how late.

That may be the internal reason that was psychological imbalanced because I wanted to complete the work quickly and no to spend more than 5 hours. That developed into a pattern of working habits unknowingly.

The author was a bit unhappy with his brothers' choice not to help for whatever reason the parents' works.

The external factors were that I was fighting to create time for studying my school homework, and the tension may have built on it eventually, I suffered migraine headache attacks! I always tried to remain calm regardless of the environment. I set a goal (tertiary education) and two objectives (aiming for a banking and finance job and savings using the method of spend below income as a habit) for my studies. (Please refer to *My Mother's Love* book (Dr Tan, 2021)). That developed my firm belief in studying smartly and self-management for health. Whenever possible, I tried to organise a timetable to guide me.

After my analysis, I adapted to organising my daily work and school homework because I needed to balance my life. But I must have enough rest without being emotionally affected by the environment that I was facing daily.

In chapters 1 and 2, I shared with my readers that in the bank, we were short-handed by calling the attention of the human resource manager. The messenger delivering the documents was always not around, but the human resource manager could not do anything. That was the circumstance in 1978. And it resulted in me suffering migraine. The doctor changed my migraine prescription to Pons tan and Cafe got. These medicines have addictive side effects, and a vicious cycle becomes a reality.

Upgrading Myself through Further Studies – A Promise to My Late Father and Mother

The author's commitment to his father was to further his study and find time to fulfil that goal. The author graduated from the University of Western Australia as doctor of business administration after completing his MBA (Distinction, Strategic Marketing, Hull, UK) in 1994.

Later, I continued with my doctoral degree researching the model of propensity to stay of Chartered Accountants with 367 samples supported by six Public Accounting Firms.

I graduated on 26 July 2019. It should have been earlier, but the arrangement of three external examiners resulted in the unpreventable delay in terms of organisation.

Dr K Tan healed my migraine on 1 March 2014 while I was doing my last part of online survey participated by six public accounting firms, the doctoral research. Therefore, the author can contribute more to Singapore at a greater height.

With the treatments and consultation of my migraine headache attacks with Dr K Tan of NNI Clinic in the government hospital, I recovered to my goal of healthiness.

Dr K Tan is careful in checking and is a committed neurologist, and finally, on 1 March 2014, I fully recovered.

Today my migraine recovery is already seven years since I requested Dr K Tan to allow an interval for me to be confident and not too dependent on RELPAX. I am confident today without taking REPLEX since 1 March 2014. The coming consultation is fixed in April 2022, and I will ask Dr K Tan to allow me an open date for future because I wanted to totally discharge from my diary recording.

Organisation and Development of Works Based on Adequate Rest of Brain

The author promised himself not to overwork because the stress may result in recurring adverse effects.

One cannot depend on doctors to improve one's health.

The author must love his banking and finance works but manage them nicely without completing the assignments.

The author chooses his relationship managers who manage their works and assignments on lending activities. One of the critical parts of the banking lending works will be present in the credit committee every Monday. Still, the credit proposal(s) must be ring-fenced all negative to become positive proposal(s).

The author discussed with his relationship managers that they should feel proud of their works under his supervision.

That was, the author promised himself as a responsible self-motivation not to invoke my migraine headache attacks (Giffin NJ et al.,2016).

The author had his rehearsal once the credit analysis was ready for presentation to the chairperson at the credit committee.

The author recovered on 1 March 2014. Although there were many delays, it was still within his goal.

Monitor the Intake of Pons tan and Cafe got Not to Overdose

In 1978, the main issue that triggered my migraine was that the messengers were not doing their work correctly.

The author requested the human resource manager of the mid-size American bank to put up a routine roster for them. As the head, the author managed getting the deal completed without errors.

That was my professional responsibility.

If they were not around to send the foreign exchange deal report to the foreign exchange division, the bank would be held responsible and would have a lousy service name, not to mention the loss. The author made it clear in a memo to the employee that his department would not be accountable.

In the fluctuating foreign markets, it was terrible to have unreliable service. We had to take responsibility. That would have improved or reduced my migraine attacks.

Conclusion

The author's migraine came from the stress of overwork on the job.

However, it is the author's love career because that is his professional life preference in that transformation.

The author initially had significantly more significant reductions in migraine headache pain intensity in less than one hour, taking the acetaminophen, aspirin, and caffeine combination (Giffin et al., 2016; Burstein R, 2000) in February 1978.

The author had never taken sick leaves because of migraine.

Unfortunately, because of heavy-loaded work at the bank, the attacks became more frequent and resulted in the bank's doctor's prescription of Pons tan and Cafe got.

I requested the duty memo to all messengers with acknowledgement because they were in the bank to work, but they were not doing anything to fulfil their responsibility of leaving no stone unturned.

I shared with you in chapter 2 the symptoms of my migraine attacks, such as stiffness of my right hand and pains on the right side of the neck and right eye (the worst because it was like a needle poking on the right eye).

My method of detection of the symptoms will prevent me from being able to work efficiently.

Thus, at levels 4–5, I would take pons tan and café got before April 2002 to keep migraine attacks at bay.

I did not want migraine attacks to occur.

The sharp pain in the author's right eye caused significant discomfort, but the headaches were the worst of all. However, the author was confident that it was only a matter of time for Dr

K Tan to heal him completely. He also consumed a lot of foods rich in antioxidants, like tomatoes, watermelons, cucumbers, and apples. We shall proceed further in Chapter 8 to raveling the torturing of serve migraine for 36 years.

Chapter 8

Tortured by Severe Migraine for 36 Years

Managing My 36-year Migraine up to My Recovery on 1 March 2014

From here on, I will use *I* instead of *the author*.

After entering a banking and finance career, I had been facing the challenges of headaches since 2 January 1978.

After 1 February 1978, it turned into a migraine headache acknowledging short-handed because the messengers always disappeared to send foreign exchange reporting papers to the Treasury Division.

I discussed the issue with the human resource manager to develop a duty list that would prevent them from disappearing.

Later a local bank called me via a friend to join its international banking division. So I left the midsize American bank without other considerations.

The local bank did not have such a problem.

The problem is the size of the bank.

I stayed at the bank for a short while. One large American bank headhunted me to market financial service products like travellers' cheques to banks. I built my contacts with banks for that relatively short period. My migraine attacks did not happen during that time, less than a year. It looked like my migraine attacks had some psychological effects.

Then one day I met a head of Bank of America's Travellers' Cheques Division. He tried to convince me to take on the offer, and I rejected it, but he continued to justify the size of the bank as crucial and of paramount importance. The total package, including salary, was acceptable to me. I was convinced to join them on the marketing side of the bank's Travellers' Cheques Division. That was on 1 August 1981.

The culture of the bank was very different. Because I was on the marketing side, many services needed to go through the operations side. After a year there, I did not feel I was at the right place, although the position as an assistant manager in those early days sounded acceptable. I did not want to work in that unconducive environment. Another prominent American bank offered and asked me to head its import trade finance department in the trade finance division. Because of the reputation of the bank. I joined them as assistant manager.

That was on 1 August 1982. This bank's culture was suitable for me. The bank selected me to coordinate a commercial and retail loans system (CARLS) project. After the project succeeded on 6 September 1984, On 6 September 1985, the American bank decided to send me to attend the Asia Pacific area's operations management development (OMD) programme in Hong Kong for three months ending on 6 December 1985. There, I met different country managers and made friends from Asia and the USA. There were 35 participants. All were helpful, but a few, like the Japanese and the Taiwanese, needed help to improve their English project papers. They asked me, and I helped them improve their proposal for their projects.

The migraine attacks occurred on alternate days, and I considered it an improvement. So I recorded down the triggers. I recorded every occurrence in Hong Kong. I focused on detecting the real causes. By the end of the project, on 6 December 1985, my mum, my wife, and my two sons joined me in Hong Kong for a week. After coordinating the CARLS project in Singapore main office, it yielded positive results, and we put the project operational on 6 September 1984.

When I attended the Asia Pacific area's operation management development programme, I stayed at Elizabeth Apartment in Causeway Bay. The programme was not easy. We needed to present a credit analysis in the programme, which I aimed for according to my goal and two objectives (My Mother's Love (Dr Tan, 2021) discussed in chapter 7.

Singapore Central Bank (also known as the Monetary Authority of Singapore), in 2000, encouraged the mergers of Singapore banks.

A local bank convinced me to join a larger Singapore bank, where I became head of a team in SME for two years. The bank started to have a project on re-engineering credit management programme. After successfully coordinating the credit management project reengineering, the bank transferred me to the corporate banking division as head of a team doing larger and structured financings, including syndications of loans and commodities financings. The biggest was aircraft financing for a reputable airline. The borrower convinced the bank to use a subsidiary in Hong Kong to invest US$5 million as equity while the loan is under syndication. That was in December 1992.

I was not able to join the borrower in Seattle to see the delivery of the aircraft. The migraine attacks became more frequent. I was concerned about the medicines I was prescribed, Pons tan and Cafe got, and I could not overdose as advised by the bank's panel of doctors. However, it turned into an unwelcome vicious cycle. Shortly after, I consulted the doctors on Pons tan and Cafe got medicines. The goal was to protect me from the vicious cycle that I did not want. The doctor told me that Pons tan and Cafe got are pain killers, and overdosage is harmful.

Later, in February 1997, a foreign bank headhunted me as head of corporate banking. I did aircraft engines financing on syndications of loan structure for a reputable airline company. However, in 1999, I felt that the bank could not understand the transferable loan facility, a hybrid structure involving loans and corporate finance.

My friend called me to join its banking group. I decided to join them as the group head of SME and structured trade finance.

My migraine attacks were my concerns.

In June/July 1997, the first Asian financial crisis hit, and it badly affected banking sector. I saw liquidity problems taking place in some banks.

The government and the Singapore Central Bank encouraged the merger of Singapore banks to become larger and more robust. The Singapore Central Bank boosted merger had its reasons. OCBC Bank bought Keppel TatLee Bank in June 2001, and United Overseas Bank bought Overseas Union Bank in September 2001. I viewed the merger activities as

Singapore Central Bank's move to promote Singapore as a solid global financial centre.

Have discipline not to always depend/ overdose on Pons tan and Cafe got

My already-severe migraine was getting worse. Their daily occurrence worried me the most. After taking Pons tan and Cafe got, within five to ten minutes, it would let up, and I continued working without needing to take a sick leave. I did not want the migraine to affect my productivity.

Arranging a Routine, Record-Keeping, and Knowing the Side Effects of RELPAX

In March 2002, I could no longer stop the pains and stiffness on my right hand. Thus, I discussed my situation with my wife. She agreed that I should tender my resignation. I resigned when OCBC Bank merged with Keppel TatLee Bank. I then set up my asset management company. And I still needed a doctor. A friend introduced me to a migraine specialist at a private hospital. The doctor advised that I should not be dependent on Pons tan and Cafe got. He recommended hospitalisation for four days to have dripping procedures to get out of the dependency on the medicines. That hospitalisation cost me a few thousands of dollars, but it did not work for me. The doctor then prescribed RELPAX, an expensive Pfizer product.

My friend suggested going to a government hospital's NNI Clinic's too see a neurologist, and the treatments would be under subsidies. In April 2002, I started seeing Dr K Tan at the NNI Clinic. After consultation, Dr K Tan said to use

RELPAX. Although it was expensive, I had to try it. But I must discipline myself not to overdose. During the first consultations and treatments, Dr K Tan asked me to be more vigilant not to take RELPAX every day, even if the daily occurrence seemed unfriendly to me. From that day on, Dr K Tan would see me every three months. I set up a recording system on my routine. The goal was to stop the migraine attacks. I continued to take antioxidant fruits. My mind was firm that I must recover in 10–12 years from April 2002.

What will be the consequences of overdosing on RELPAX?

It was explained in chapter 5 that migraine is a costly illness and it has risk and fear factors. RELPAX is for adults who suffer from migraine. RELPAX has the antimigraine medication El triptan. Adults who suffer from migraine must be cautious in taking triptans as it narrows swollen blood vessels in the patient's brain, creating less pain. Hence, the risk of overdosage is high. It comes in 20mg and 40mg tablets. After taking a pill and the symptoms did not let up, another pill can be taken only after two hours. Although I did not have that experience, the more common side effects of RELPAX are as follows:

Feeling weak
Sleepiness
Tightness and pains

Following the list above, patients are not supposed to overdose. Listen to your doctor's instructions.

Disciple myself not to overdose despite the daily occurrence of migraine attacks

My migraine was severe, and I was cautious not to overdose. I pray for God's blessing to heal this migraine so I can share my knowledge and contribute to Singapore's banking and finance sector to support the Singapore government's ambitions of helping and training other countries as well.

I read more books on antioxidant fruits as a supplement to reduce tensions.

Because overdosage is harmful, I started taking a lot of fruits that are high in antioxidants. I have preference to four fruits that I think are helpful to me: tomatoes, watermelons, cucumbers, and apples.

The study of Mood and migraine relationship

I will try not to be emotional always because the study's findings that there is a relationship between mood and migraine. That was the reason Dr K Tan suggested to be calm, avoiding mood or emotion to take place. I also practice not to over work and work under stress. I love my banking and finance works.

A survey of thirty thousand plus participants in a Canadian study, showed that major depression, bipolar disorder, and social phobia were all at least twice as prevalent in migraine subjects. The findings were not in demographic and socioeconomic variables (Fanning et al., 2012

Hence, it was not independent of mood (dry crying internally to some migraine patients because of pains), headache patients and spirit appeared essential in migraine headache attack patients (Bolay H et al., 2002; Burstein R, et al., 2000).

Fatigue and Arousal in Migraine

Migraine had tortured the author since 1 February 1978. Migraine attacks were unkind to the author. I, the author, not only suffered from migraine pains but also fatigue as a vague and multifactorial symptom.

As a migraine patient, I must consider everything or relationship. Although fatigue is different, it has interaction between them and a general difficulty among patients distinguishing from a dominant feature of migraines (migraine headaches and more recently, researchers found the associations with sleep disorders (Buse DC et al., 2012).

Conclusion

The happiest event since 1 February 1978 was on 1 March 2014, when my neurologist Dr K Tan completely healed my migraine with his knowledge, skills, and patience. That day was memorable because I did not take RELPAX until today, which is a lapse of eight years. I am happy and relax in relationship to migraine, but I continue to take the four types of fruits (Tomatoes, Watermelons. Apples, and cucumbers).

That is not mood, but I have 95% level of confidence with Dr K Tan. However, I will consult Dr K Tan for an open date of appointment in the future.

I am more inclined to be positive on my healing by Dr K Tan on 1 March 2014, and I was all right. Therefore, it was finally free from migraines after thirty-six years!

Dr K Tan is understanding, knowledgeable, skillful, and communicates patiently.

A big thank you to Dr K Tan!

The brand RELPAX is a product of Pfizer. It has El triptan hydrobromide. It is expensive without government subsidy as it costs S$10 apiece. Hence, I was cautious about its side effects.

I was thankful to my friend who recommended that I visit NNI Clinic to see the neurologist Dr K Tan. The healing of my migraine was worth celebrating. My life has changed, and I am free. It is the quality of life that I have been looking for since 1 February 1978. The conclusion on chapter 9 discloses the wisdom of managing risk, fear, and push up confidence with motivation internally.

Chapter 9

My Quality of Life Began on the healing of my migraine on 1 March 2014 by Dr K Tan

On 1 March 2014, my freedom-from-pain day, I fully recovered from my 36-year migraine, thanks to my neurologist Dr K Tan.

The Open Sky's My Limit in My Banking-and-Finance, Asset Management Career

Nothing can compare to a full recovery from a 36-year migraine. The nightmare was over, and I would not let it return. I was so encouraged and happy. Money cannot buy my full recovery from migraine. For now, the sky is a limit to me, and I wanted to repay my tertiary education. Without the education and training, I would not be bilingual, speaking excellently in English and Mandarin. It was God's blessing that a friend convinced me to consult with and be treated by Dr K Tan of NNI Clinic in a government hospital.

When I set up my asset management firm, I continued to contribute to Asia by training bankers in Malaysia, Indonesia, China, and Hong Kong. Although the environment may be changing because of COVID-19, there are unpredictable and uncertain changes in the climate, it is meaningful in contribute knowledge in banking and finance to bankers in the APR area, helping Asian banks be more assertive in managing people's wealth honestly.

More Contributions to Singapore If My Migraine Healed

I will continue contributing to Singapore by sharing knowledge and skills in managing banking and finance transactions by training banks' executives and managers. Although we are in the midst of a pandemic brought about by COVID-19, that is the goal of getting Singapore to progress steadily. We can use online technological platforms to share our experience and knowledge with Singaporeans.

Sharing the Author's Experience and Management of the Costly Illness

I wanted to share my third book in 2021 to inspire my readers to be more productive, and free from migraines by consulting a neurologist doctor.

We are in third to fourth positions of the global financial centre, with the reputation of well regulations in place to guide and protect Singapore's global financial centre status.

From the 1997/1998 Asian financial crisis, the Singapore government learned to set policies to guide Singapore's advancement. The government called upon me to collaborate with the World Bank trainers to help the People's Bank of China to train senior bankers on credit risk management and case studies.

Despite my migraine, I supported the Monetary Authority of Singapore. The chairman of the People's Bank of China, China's central bank, requested that I use Putonghua for training to lead direct input without an interpreter.

I asked the World Bank that the request should be accommodated, which they did not answer me direct. They said that there was no prohibition on this. I went ahead of the request with success and happiness of all the senior banker-participants. I prepared the notes in English as instructed. The senior bankers were happy. Thank goodness, I had no migraine attacks.

Freedom of a long-awaited quality of life andfamily members

I had never celebrated a birthday before, and I took 1 March 2014 as my birthday celebration. I looked forward to my recovery from migraine. There were signals, and I awaited the improvements of my migraine because there were no headaches for a few days.

I shared my feelings, my inspiration for recovery, with Dr K Tan. I was excited for this to happen to change my life with the quality that I await 36 years.

The New Journey Begins to See a New Horizon

I have been taking antioxidant fruits and vegetables for years. I read loads of books about antioxidant fruits and vegetables for my goal of no migraine with REPLAX until I am healed.

On 1 March 2014, the tightness and pain of my right hand led me to use tomato, cut in two pieces, and rub it on my right hand while I was preparing my doctoral thesis. After rubbing for one hour, a miracle happened: My right hand's stiffness disappeared unexpectedly.

So I used the other half of the tomato to rub on my forehead's tightness. The process took about one hour, and the tightness disappeared as well; my head was like a baby's head, without tightness or stress. I did not take RELPAX, and it did not get worse. This improvement gave me confidence. And I reported it to Dr K Tan in our next consultation.

Sharing My Life after Recovery from Migraine with Reader Patients

On my next visit to the hospital, on the appointment date, I must share my joy on my total recovery from migraine with Dr K Tan. It was on 1 March 2014, an excellent day in my life, and I was free of migraine. I thanked Dr K Tan and promised him that I would author a book to share my migraine experience.

Self-Discipline and Development in Health and Wealth (Savings and Investments)

Because of inflation, CPF savings would be inadequate for anyone's retirement. It is crystal-clear to have disciple of spending below the income. The Warren Buffett's philosophy and value investing method.

Beginning in 1985, encouraged by my colleague

While I was at the premium American bank's main office in Singapore, my colleague told me to cultivate investment ability, applying my rich knowledge of finance and accounting to my advantage against inflation. The CPF savings will not be enough for our retirement funds.

I told him to invest in the property markets because inflation is an international symptom. I was preserving asset value and having savings to invest in the property. That was during the first Asian financial crisis. He invested in a government condominium known as HUDC. After holding for two years, he sold at and had a yield of 20% before he bought a new private condominium for four days for reinvestment. Now my life has changed, and I have freedom of life in terms of quality recovering from migraine. I distanced myself from the medicines because I wanted to cut the fear.

Conclusion

Costly illness and risk and fear factors

Chapter 5 discussed costly illness and risk and fear factors. I shared the risk and fear factors as an individual's health is a priority because fitness becomes essential. Because of this, fatigue is a vague and multifactorial symptom, which might affect sleep and arousal, systemic health, mood, and other exogenous factors, including medications. The author shares his experience fighting migraine headaches (Giffin NJ et al.,

2016; Steiner TJ et al., 2018), and the author wanted to find out the reasons to overcome the risk and fear factors. In contrast, fatigue is a dominant feature of migraine.

Threats of Migraine

One of the threats of migraine is that it may affect the patients' careers. Although the author managed well and he refused to take sick leaves, the author faced not only financial stress but also risks and fears brought about by migraine. The author took RELPAX to manage pains that affected the quality of his life, which was very unhealthy.

Health and Healthcare and Wealth

The relationship between health and healthcare are closely associated with wealth Furthermore, it may affect the individual's career development. Hence, curing migraine is always a first priority for any individual.

Healthy body will have healthy and happy career horizon. It is the quality of life that is critical to any individual. As an illness management, the individual sufferers should not allow the mood to come into the horizon of migraine patients.

I made the research on fruits for many years because I read those books written by medical backgrounds authors. I have the inclination to take fruits for health reasons. The reasons why I take many fruits are owing to fruits are not harmful to a human body. They can also perform detoxification function.

RELPAX is no longer in my mind today. I also drink about 10 cups of water every day.

The most happiness that I acquired after my recovery of migraine on 1 March 2014 is the quality of life I have been looking forwards. Hence, health and healthcare are my priority. I want a happy family in which I will continue to be enjoying playing with my three grandchildren. That is the quality of life.

Another observation is that I will take rest earlier every night and stop typing of my work by six o'clock in the evening and proceed to take my dinner.

Continue my Contributions to Singapore in the areas of Banking and Finance, and Asset Management Investments

It was an encouragement to have my migraines healed by Dr K Tan on 1 March 2014 because I have a strong inclination of Dr K Tan's treatment processes, pain management, and consultation advice.

I shared with Dr K Tan on every consultation and my improvements on my calmness to not overdoses of RELPAX.

Dr K Tan was very patience listening each consultation and recorded my progress improvement on his computer recording my migraine improvements.

Open Horizon for me After Healing of Migraines on 1 March 2014

From April 2002 when Dr K Tan diagnosed me each time, he was happy of my discipline on not overdosing on RELPAX. That discipline, Dr K Tan commented that I should be able to heal my migraines I a few years. That encouragement is very positive.

After I completed my first book on 'My Mother's Love', my confidence for future appeared strong and positive. My mood has been getting better that gives me more confidence. As such, I decided to discuss with Dr K Tan to allow me an open date for future appointments because I did not take RELPAX after 1 March 2014. I have full confidence with regard to migraine. It is a distance from me.

The horizon of life is under control management for my quality of life. Hence, sky is a limit to me after migraine recovery. I am patience enough to have eight years for me to have that 95% level of confidence.

I completed two books in 2021 – "My Mother's Love." They have correlations to this book.

Dr K Tan Healed My Migraine on 1 March 2014

I am completely all right after recovering from migraine 8 years ago. I salute and thank Dr K Tan for encouraging me to author this book on my recovery that I discussed with him after my migraine recovery on 1 March 2014. The quality of life I was looking forwards that fulfilled without emotional factors. I am happy that I could contribute to Singapore in banking and finance, and asset management investments and wealth management are beyond expectation.

Thanks for readers' support of this book

I thank readers in wanting to heal your migraine in that you may have learned my disciple to have a goal of healing my 36 years of migraine. A big thank you!

Appendix

Diagram on level of pains advised by the doctor that I can decide to take the migraine medicines on time to stop the migraine attacks and develop an elevated level of pains.

References

Afridi, S K; Kaube, H; and Goadsby, P J. "Glyceryl trinitrate triggers premonitory symptoms in migraineurs." Pain. 2004; 110: 675–680.

Ashina, M; Hansen, J M; A′ Dunga, B O; et al. Human models of migraine – short-term pain for long-term gain. Nat Rev Neurol 2017; 13: 713–724.

Ashkenazi, A; Silberstein, S; Jakubowski, M; and Burstein, R. "Improved identification of allodynic migraine patients using a questionnaire." Cephalalgia. 2007;27:325–329. [PMC free article] [PubMed] [Google Scholar]

Blau, J N. Adult migraine: the patient observed. In: Blau, J N, editor. Migraine – Clinical, therapeutic, conceptual and research aspects. Chapman and Hall Ltd; Cambridge: 1987. pp. 3–30. [Google Scholar]

Blau, J N and Dexter, S L. "The site of pain origin during migraine attacks." Cephalalgia. 1981;1:143–147. [PubMed] [Google Scholar]

Blooded, L M; Stokes, M; Buse, D C; et al (2012) Cost of healthcare for patients with migraine in five European countries: Results from the international burden of migraine study (IBMS). J Headache Pain. 13:361–378.

Bolay, H; Reuter, U; Dunn, A K; Huang, Z; Boas, D A; and Moskowitz, M A. "Intrinsic brain activity triggers trigeminal meningeal afferents in a migraine model." Nat Med. 2002;8:136–142. [PubMed] [Google Scholar]

Bose, P; Karsan, N; and Goadsby, P J. Migraine Is More Than Just Headache: Is the Link to Chronic Fatigue and Mood Disorders Simply Due to Shared Biological Systems? PMID: 34149377, PMCID: PMC8209296, DOI: 10.3389/fnhum.2021.646692, 2021.

Boyer, J and Liu, R H. "Apple phytochemicals and their health benefits." Nutrition Journal. 2004 vol 3, no 5.

Bullock, R, PhD. Human Neural Stem Cells: A New Approach to Restorative Therapy for Severe Traumatic Brain Injury, University of Miami Miller School of Medicine. 2019.

Burstein, R. "Deconstructing migraine headache into peripheral and central sensitization." Pain. 2001; 89:107–110. [PubMed] [Google Scholar]

Burstein, R; Cutrer, F M; and Yarnitsky, D. "The development of cutaneous allodynia during a migraine attack: Clinical evidence for the sequential recruitment of spinal and supraspinal nociceptive neurons in migraine." Brain. 2000;123:1703–1709. [PubMed] [Google Scholar]

Buse, D C; Manack, A N; Fanning, K M; et al (2012) Chronic migraine prevalence, disability, and sociodemographic factors: Results from the American migraine prevalence and prevention study. Headache 52(10):1456–1470.

Christiansen, I; Thomsen, L L; Daugaard, D; et al. "Glyceryl trinitrate induces attacks of migraine without aura in sufferers of migraine with aura." Cephalalgia. 1999;19:660–667, discussion p. 26.

Giffin, N J; Lipton, R B; Silberstein, S D, et al. The migraine postdrome: An electronic diary study. Neurology 2016; 87: 309–313.

Goschorska, M; Gutowska, I; Barnowska-Bosiacka, I: Barczak, K; and Chlubek, D. 2017, The Use of Antioxidants in the Treatment of Migraine, PMID: 32012936 PMCID: PMC7070237 DOI: 10.3390/antiox9020116

Headache Classification Committee of the International Headache Society. The International Classification of Headache Disorders, third edition (beta version). Cephalalgia 2013; 33: 629–808.

Karsan, N; and Goadsby, P J. 2021, Migraine Is More Than Just Headache: Is the Link to Chronic Fatigue and Mood Disorders Simply Due to Shared Biological Systems? PMCID: 34149377; PMCID: PMC8209296; DOI: 10.3389/fnhum.2021.646692.

Karsan, N; Bose, P; and Goadsby, P J. The migraine premonitory phase. Continuum 2018; 24: 996–1008.

Merriam-Webster's Unabridged Dictionary.

Newman, J; Karsan, N; Thompson, C, et al. "Comparing postdrome and premonitory symptoms to self-reported triggers in spontaneous and nitroglycerin (NTG)-triggered migraine attacks." Cephalalgia. 2019; 39: 282–283.

Ong, J J Y; Patnaik, D; YC Chan1; Oliver Simon4; and Finkelstein, E A. 2020. Economic burden of migraine in Singapore, Cephalalgia Reports, Volume 3: 1–1, Sage, Corresponding author: Jonathan Jia Yuan Ong, Division of Neurology, Department of Medicine, National University Hospital, National University Health System, 1E Kent Ridge Road, NUHS Tower Block, Singapore 119228.

Payne, K A; Varon, S F; Kawata, A K; et al. "The international burden of migraine study (IBMS): Study design, methodology, and baseline cohort characteristics." Cephalalgia. 2011:31(10):1116–1130.

Peres et al. The Journal of Headache and Pain. 2017:18:37 DOI 10.1186/s10194-017-0742-fremanezumab-vfrm injection, 2018 CGRP Monoclonal Antibodies John P. Cunha, RxList DO, FACOEP, RxList.

Saper, Joel R, MD and Magee, Kenneth R, MD. Revised and Updated Freedom from Headaches, Simon & Schuster, Inc. 1981.

Schulte, L H; Jurgens, T P; and May, A. Photo-, osmo- and phonophobia in the premonitory phase of migraine: Mistaking symptoms for triggers? J Headache Pain 2015; 16: 14.

Steiner, T J; Sovner, L J; Vos, T; Jensen, R; and Katsarava, Z. (2018) Migraine is first cause of disability in under 50s: Will health politicians now take notice? J Headache Pain 19:17.

Tan, S K. 2019. "Factors Affecting Chartered Accountants' Propensity to Stay in Singapore Public Accounting Firms." Doctoral Thesis, University of Western Australia.

Tan, 2021. My Mother's Love – Growing My Life from Zero to Life Success Like Dr Jack Tan, www.partridgepublishing. com/singapore.

Thomsen, L L; Kruuse, C; Iversen, H K; et al. A nitric oxide donor (nitroglycerin) triggers genuine migraine attack. Eur J Neurol 1994; 1: 73–80.

Togha, M; Jahromi, S R; Ghorbani, Z; Ghaemi, A; and Rafiee, P. 2019. "An investigation of oxidant/antioxidant balance in patients with migraine: A case-control study," BMC Neurology volume 19, Article number: 323 (2019) Cite this article, 2271 Accesses, 10 Citations,1 Altmetric Metricsdetails.

Vos, T; Allen, C; Arora, M; Barber, R M; Bhutta, Z A; Brown, A; et al (2016) Global, regional, and national incidence, prevalence, and years lived with disability for 310 diseases and injuries, 1990–2015: A systematic analysis for the global burden of disease study 2015. Lancet 388:1545–1602.

Jia and Wang, 2021, "Introductory Chapter: Studies on Cucumber", Reviewed: 22 March 2021 Published: 8 May 2021, DOI: 10.5772/intechopen.97360.